PHOTOGRAPHY-BASED APPROACHES IN HEALTH RESEARCH

This groundbreaking guide introduces health researchers and students to innovative photography-based research methods in healthcare, capitalising on photographic techniques' advantages over traditional approaches. The book provides a structured framework currently lacking in healthcare research, offering comprehensive guidance for navigating this emerging methodological landscape.

Photography-Based Approaches in Health Research: Techniques and Applications explores diverse photography-based methodologies, including photo-elicitation, photovoice, visual ethnography, photographic collage, and photo-storytelling. It examines the interconnection between photography and phenomenology in health research, providing historical context while exploring future developments in artificial intelligence applications. Authentic case studies from the author's mental health research and lived experience enhance real-world applicability, while the final chapter offers practical exercises for immediate application. A dedicated chapter addresses the complex ethical considerations inherent in photographic research methods.

This essential resource serves health researchers, graduate students, and academics in public health, nursing, medicine, psychology, and health and allied professions. The practical guidance for planning, designing, and conducting photography-based research makes it invaluable for qualitative researchers, visual methodologists, and anyone seeking to integrate visual and textual data in healthcare and well-being studies, offering clear frameworks for formulating research questions, collecting and analysing data, and reporting findings.

Dr Lucian Hadrian Milasan is a senior lecturer in mental health nursing and a qualitative researcher at Nottingham Trent University (the Institute of Health and Allied Professions), where he teaches and contributes to mental health practice and research modules at both undergraduate and postgraduate levels.

PHOTOGRAPHY-BASED APPROACHES IN HEALTH RESEARCH

Techniques and Applications

Lucian Hadrian Milasan

Routledge
Taylor & Francis Group
LONDON AND NEW YORK

Designed cover image: Getty Images @RasikaSekhara

First published 2026
by Routledge
4 Park Square, Milton Park, Abingdon, Oxon OX14 4RN

and by Routledge
605 Third Avenue, New York, NY 10158

Routledge is an imprint of the Taylor & Francis Group, an informa business

British Library Cataloguing-in-Publication Data
A catalogue record for this book is available from the British Library

ISBN: 978-1-032-88396-0 (hbk)
ISBN: 978-1-032-87727-3 (pbk)
ISBN: 978-1-003-53754-0 (ebk)

DOI: 10.4324/9781003537540

Typeset in Times New Roman
by Apex CoVantage, LLC

CONTENTS

FIGURES

TABLES

ABOUT THE AUTHOR

Dr Lucian Hadrian Milasan is a senior lecturer in mental health nursing at Nottingham Trent University (the Institute of Health and Allied Professions), where he teaches and contributes to mental health practice and research modules at both undergraduate and postgraduate levels. He is a visual and qualitative researcher with a strong focus on lived experiences of mental distress and mental health recovery. Dr Milasan specialises in integrating photography-based methods such as photo-elicitation and photovoice with qualitative approaches, particularly phenomenology and post-phenomenology. His research portfolio in this area is steadily expanding and includes a systematic review on the use of photography in mental health research (Milasan et al., 2022); cultural explorations of experiences and meanings of recovery and resilience (Milasan, 2023; Milasan & Finta, 2025); and a methodological article on the therapeutic benefits of photography as a research tool (Milasan, 2024a), to name only a few. He has also authored several book chapters, including work on photo-elicitation in healthcare research (Milasan, 2022) and an exploration of artificial intelligence in phototherapy and therapeutic photogrphy (Milasan, 2026). Currently, Dr Milasan is investigating the evolution of visual and photographic research methods in the context of emerging technologies such as artificial intelligence (Milasan, 2024b) – work that contributes to a contemporary understanding of photography as a research method within a rapidly advancing digital landscape. Committed to producing accessible, innovative, and inspiring scholarship, Dr Milasan continues to publish work that informs academics, health practitioners, researchers, and students across health and allied professions.

Selection of author's works

Milasan, L. H. (2022). Photo-elicitation: Unleashing imagery in healthcare research. In K. Hinsliff-Smith, McGarry, J., & Ali, P. (Eds.), *Arts based health care research: A multidisciplinary perspective* (pp. 51–67). Springer. https://link.springer.com/chapter/10.1007/978-3-030-94423-0_5

Milasan, L. H. (2023). "Mending fractured personalities": A photography-based cultural study of recovery from mental distress in Romania. *Transcultural Psychiatry, 60*(2), 226–243. https://doi.org/10.1177/13634615221119373

Milasan, L. H. (2024a). 'Taking pictures is like treasure hunting': Exploring the therapeutic value of photography as a qualitative research method. *International Journal of Qualitative Methods, 23*. https://doi.org/10.1177/16094069241236219

Milasan, L. H. (2024b). Unveiling the transformative potential of Ai-generated imagery in enriching mental health research. *Qualitative Health Research, 35*(14), 1527–1535. https://doi.org/10.1177/10497323241274767

Milasan, L. H. (2026, in press). Phototherapy, therapeutic photography and AI. In D. Lowenthal (Ed.), *Phototherapy and therapeutic photography in a digital age* (2nd ed.). Routledge.

Milasan, L. H., Bingley, A. F., & Fisher, N. R. (2022). The big picture of recovery: A systematic review on the evidence of photography-based methods in researching recovery from mental distress. *Arts & Health, 14*(2), 165–185. https://doi.org/10.1080/17533015.2020.1855453

Milasan, L. H., & Finta, O. (2025). "Rising like Phoenix from the ashes": An arts-based qualitative study of mental health resilience and recovery in Romania. *Qualitative Health Research* [e-pub]. https://doi.org/10.1177/10497323251355120

ACKNOWLEDGEMENTS

This book was born from the light and shadows of my photographic journey – therapeutic and research – and from the voices of those who walked beside me, people who opened my eyes to photography not only as an art but also as a language of healing and inquiry. Some of these people remain concealed behind pseudonyms, yet their presence lingers in every page. To them, I offer my deepest gratitude.

I am indebted to the ambassadors of photography at the Estuar Foundation who contributed to this book with their creations – Laura, Rodion, Călin, Mihai, Robert, and Judit – guided with care by Orsolya Finta, social worker and manager of the Day Centre in Cluj-Napoca, Romania – a hub of creativity and healing. It was there that my own journey began with my first photography group that showed me the value of photography not only for aesthetics and technical skills but also as a way to open doors to meaning, connection, and transformation.

My thanks extend to my colleagues at the Institute of Health and Allied Professions at Nottingham Trent University. I want to particularly thank Prof Jayne Brown, whose mentorship and wisdom shaped the path that led me to bring photography back to the heart of my research. I would also like to add here many thanks to Prof Del Lowenthal – Emeritus Professor of Psychotherapy and Counselling at the University of Roehampton, London – for his foreword and his inspiring work on the therapeutic power of photography.

Writing this book was a rollercoaster with its highs and lows, with days oozing with ideas and days when pages were staring blankly at me. I am fortunate to be surrounded by family and friends who reminded me of the worth of this work, even when I could not see it myself. I would like to thank my nephew, Nicholas, for his visual contributions that hopefully opened his appetite for photography. And a special thanks to Craig, my steadfast listener and support through life's many storms.

Last but not least, I would like to thank my faithful companion, Freya, a welcome distraction who ensured I take regular screen breaks. She agreed with a bark to let some of her pictures appear in this book in exchange for a handful of her favourite treats.

FOREWORD

When I first saw the proposal for this book, I was immediately taken, which is not my usual experience, with both the importance of its subject matter and its clarity.

In recent years, we have witnessed a growing acknowledgement – both within psychotherapy and the wider field of health research – that not all experience can be adequately grasped through words alone. Much of what matters in human suffering, care, and recovery is tacit, embodied, and pre-reflective. Photography, with its capacity to arrest a moment while simultaneously revealing what exceeds representation, offers a distinctive way of approaching these dimensions. It is therefore a pleasure to introduce this book – *Photography-Based Approaches in Health Research: Techniques and Applications* – which brings together a thoughtful and comprehensive account of how images can deepen our understanding of health, illness, and the human condition.

My own work in therapeutic photography and critical practice has long been concerned with the ways in which visual methods can make present what is ordinarily marginalised in research: the unspoken, the affective, and the relational. What we often find, whether in therapeutic encounters or other research contexts, is that photographs open a different kind of dialogue – one that situates meaning not only in narratives but also in textures, atmospheres, and the ambiguities that resist tidy interpretation. This book recognises that potential and provides a rigorous framework for working with such complexity. Furthermore, here we can see photographic research as methods in their own right and not just as important adjuncts to the more standard non-visual approaches.

Importantly, Dr Milasan does not present photography as a neutral or purely technical tool. Instead, the book situates photographic methods within philosophical and ethical considerations important for any researcher working in healthcare. The chapter on philosophical underpinnings and historical evolution of photography as a research method is particularly significant. It reminds us that to use photography in research is not merely to collect data but to enter into a relationship – often asymmetrical – with participants, their images, and their lived realities. The ethical chapter of this book is therefore not an add-on; it is integral to the work.

Photography-based approaches are also shown here to have therapeutic relevance. Whether through photovoice with marginalised communities, photo-elicitation in clinical settings, or participatory visual ethnography, images often allow participants to express experiences that may have been difficult to articulate verbally. Importantly, I do not advocate the therapeutic use of photographs when not facilitated by a trained psychotherapist who has had considerable personal therapy. Yet, given those vital caveats, I do strongly agree, as advocated in this book, that photography can foster reflexivity and agency for participants and can invite researchers to confront their own assumptions about health, illness, and representation.

As someone who has also long advocated for critical reflexivity in both therapy and research, I am particularly appreciative of the emphasis in this book on the researcher's responsibility to remain alert to the potential for (mis)representation. Photographs, as constructed images, can empower, but they can also objectify; they can reveal, but they can also conceal. The chapter dealing with artificial intelligence (AI) introduces an additional layer of complexity, reminding us that the image is no longer simply captured but increasingly generated, manipulated, and algorithmically interpreted. In an era when visual technologies are becoming more pervasive, Dr Milasan's careful discussion of the methodological and ethical implications of AI is timely and necessary.

Readers will also find the final chapter extremely valuable for teaching and practice. The worked examples, exercises, and applied activities offer pragmatic guidance without losing sight of the philosophical and ethical commitments that underpin the whole book. This combination of conceptual depth and practical clarity is rare and welcome.

In bringing together diverse photographic methods – photo-elicitation, photovoice, visual ethnography, photo-storytelling, and more – this book provides a unique point of reference for healthcare researchers, practitioners, and students alike. More than an instructional guide, it invites us to consider what it means to "see" in healthcare and what might become possible when we allow images to speak not just to us but with us.

It is my hope that readers will not only learn techniques from these pages but will also be encouraged to adopt a more questioning, ethically attuned, and relationally sensitive approach to photography-based research. For in the end, the value of such work lies not only in what is shown but also in the human encounters – and responsibilities – that emerge in the very looking of being.

Prof Del Loewenthal
Emeritus Professor of Psychotherapy and Counselling,
University of Roehampton, London, UK, and Chair of Southern
Association for Psychotherapy and Counselling, London, UK

INTRODUCTION

Photography-Based Approaches in Health Research: Techniques and Applications represents the culmination of a long and deeply personal journey in which photography has been my constant companion across the many roles I inhabit(ed) – student, commercial photographer, mental health professional, reviewer, healthcare educator, supervisor, researcher, and expert by experience. Photography has always been present in my life, including during my own battle with myasthenia gravis and depression – experiences that revealed the therapeutic potential of photography and inspired me to explore its role in mental health during my doctoral studies.

My PhD thesis (Milasan, 2020) highlighted a critical gap – the literature on methodological aspects of using photography in health-related research, and not only, was fragmented and inconsistent. Like many early-career and established researchers, I sought a rigorous, coherent framework for integrating photography into health research. Instead, I often encountered literature that was disjointed, incomplete, sometimes contradictory, and variable in quality and reliability. This book is my response to that challenge – a structured, evidence-informed resource for health researchers, practitioners, and students who wish to master photography as a meaningful research tool.

Aims and objectives

In this book, I aim to address this gap in the literature on using photography-based research methods in healthcare research by providing a clear and structured methodological framework that is currently lacking. The book capitalises on the advantages and methodological potential of photographic techniques (compared to traditional methods) that are increasingly used for exploring health phenomena.

The objectives that guided me throughout writing this book are:

- To explore the historical evolution and philosophical underpinnings of photography as a research method in healthcare research.
- To outline a rationale for using photographic techniques in health research by emphasising the advantages and potential they have compared to non-photographic approaches.

DOI: 10.4324/9781003537540-1

- To provide a comprehensive step-by-step guide to planning, designing, and conducting photography-based healthcare research to support health researchers and students acquire knowledge and skills in this subject area. For this purpose, the reader is guided from formulating a research question for a photographic inquiry in healthcare to making informed decisions throughout the stages of data collection and analysis, reporting findings that triangulate visual and textual data, and dissemination.
- To critically discuss ethical challenges and complexities of photographic research methods in health research, including aspects related to the use of digital technologies.
- To bridge the theoretical foundations of photographic techniques and research practice by providing authentic examples and insights into conducting photography-based research.

The book provides the reader with a comprehensive account of the most common photography-based methodologies, such as photo-elicitation, photovoice, and visual ethnography, along with less frequent uses of photography in health research, including photographic collage and digital storytelling. Historical aspects referring to the evolution of such photographic methods provide the reader with a holistic context complemented by a thought-provoking chapter on the future of photography-based research in the era of artificial intelligence.

My goal throughout this book has been to maintain a strong practical focus. For this reason, most of the chapters include comprehensive guidance for planning, designing, and conducting health research embedding photographic techniques. The practical dimension culminates in the last chapter, consisting of applications, knowledge checking, ideas for photography-based activities, and photographic outputs meant to inspire the reader. Much of the advice and many of the examples included in this book are authentic, stemming mainly from my lived experience and conducting photographic research into mental health.

Why a book on photography-based health research?

A book on the use of photography in healthcare research is important and necessary in the current context in which photography is increasingly used to enhance insights into health phenomena. Although more and more healthcare researchers utilise visual aids, there seems to be a lack of resources and clear guidance on conducting photography-based research in this subject area from a methodological and ethical perspective (Miller, 2015). Part of the problem is due to embedding photography in generic arts-based studies combining different approaches such as painting, drawing, and creative writing. In my opinion, this often leads to confusion around the benefits and methodological application of photography in research practice that may dilute the value of this approach (Milasan et al., 2022). Moreover, photography-based research studies are criticised for lacking rigour and a clear framework (Langman & Pick, 2018). This book aims to answer some essential questions that may help the reader make an informed decision on whether the use of photography, as a standalone approach, is justified and purposeful, as opposed to being an unnecessary sophistication. Furthermore, the book provides guidance on how to enhance the methodological and ethical soundness of photography-based research, particularly in healthcare.

It is known that photography can provide valuable opportunities for triangulation of research data, strengthening the methodological approaches, particularly in health areas that are difficult to articulate through textual communication and traditional research methods, for example, mental health and learning disabilities. This book capitalises on this aspect by providing a one-stop resource currently lacking on the market, guiding the audience through the often difficult-to-navigate stages of planning, designing, and conducting photography-based health research. For this purpose, questions such as "what" (is photography-based research?), "why" (is photography necessary as a research method?), and "how" (is photography-based health research conducted?) are addressed in this book. To achieve this, I draw on evidence I carefully curated to comprehensively cover content related to all the essential aspects of photography techniques in healthcare research.

Who is the book for?

To my knowledge, this is the first book exploring photographic techniques and applications in such depth with a specific focus on healthcare research. As mentioned above, the book is inspired by my own needs and struggles as a visual researcher, echoed by students and fellow researchers from health and other disciplines, for example, arts and humanities. This inspired me to align this book with the current interdisciplinary and innovative context, thinking of researchers who may wish to add photographic techniques to their methodological repertoire. At the same time, the book is also addressed to visual researchers already versed in photography as a research method who may wish to channel their expertise into health-related subjects. The latter includes researchers in arts and humanities, academics, and postgraduate research students with an interest in research combining photography and well-being on courses such as photography, digital photography, therapeutic photography, digital art and design, public art and community engagement, art and well-being, integrative arts, visual arts, media and society, and gender studies.

The book may also be appealing to health practitioners engaging in audit, service improvement, and research that may require photographic data collection and analysis. The book is also relevant to healthcare educational contexts, namely under- and postgraduate students on health-related courses such as medicine, biomedical sciences, epidemiology, public health, global health, health psychology, health research, mental health, learning disabilities, health promotion, sports and exercise sciences, environmental health, nursing, quality improvement in healthcare, and midwifery. I would also like to add allied professions courses such as art therapy, including photo-therapy and therapeutic photography, occupational therapy, paramedicine, audiology, physiotherapy, podiatry, pharmacology, nutrition, speech and language therapy, and dentistry.

Key features

Among the key features of this book, I would mention:

- Balance between the theory and practice of photography-based research methods in health-related subjects
- Focus on the benefits and challenges of using photography as a research method in healthcare
- Exploration of a wide range of photographic techniques in health research covering current and more futuristic approaches
- Processual approach to photography-based research with emphasis on hands-on experiences and practical and reflective exercises to encourage the application of theory into practice
- Accessible language aligned with a learner-centred writing style yet critical and thought-provoking.

References

Langmann, S., & Pick, D. (2018). *Photography as a social research method.* Springer.

Milasan, L. H. (2020). *Recovery snapshots: A photographic exploration of Romanian mental health service users' experience of recovery* [PhD thesis, Lancaster University]. https://eprints.lancs.ac.uk/id/eprint/149077/1/2020MilasanPhD.pdf

Milasan, L. H., Bingley, A. F., & Fisher, N. R. (2022). The big picture of recovery: A systematic review on the evidence of photography-based methods in researching recovery from mental distress. *Arts & Health, 14*(2), 165–185. https://doi.org/10.1080/17533015.2020.1855453

Miller, K. (2015). Dear critics: Addressing concerns and justifying the benefits of photography as a research method. *Social Research, 16*(3), 27. http://nbn-resolving.de/urn:nbn:de:0114-fqs1503274

1

PHOTOGRAPHY AS A RESEARCH METHOD IN HEALTHCARE

1.1 A philosophical prelude to photography

Whether approached as a research method, professional practice, hobby, artistic endeavour, or means of capturing meaningful life events, photography is deeply rooted in philosophy. Beyond serving as a physical lens through which the world can be observed, photography constitutes a source of knowledge and insight into both individual and collective perceptions of the surrounding environment and subjective life experiences.

A critical philosophical discussion of photography can be initiated by a seemingly simple question – *What is photography?* – that prompts further lines of inquiry, such as: *Is photography a form of art? Is it a technical skill? Or is it a simple representation or reflection of reality?* While scientists, philosophers, and photographers may offer different answers, undoubtedly photography extends beyond the objective documentation of reality. Photographs create rich opportunities for the production of subjective knowledge through emotional expression, creativity, and interpretation. In his seminal work *Camera Lucida*, Barthes (1993) makes a key ontological distinction between the *referent* – the actual object or scene depicted in a photograph – and *photographic signifier*, which refers to what is perceived or evoked in the viewer through reflection and introspection. Photography, therefore, can be understood as facilitating an ontological or existential journey from the immediate, concrete aspects of reality to more abstract, metaphorical, and emotionally resonant forms of expression. This interpretive journey varies depending on the degree of subjectivity or objectivity embedded in the photograph by its creator, referred to by Barthes as the *Operator*, and by how it is subsequently received by the viewer, or the *Spectator*.

For instance, a photograph of a fence (Figure 1.1) can be interpreted literally as a physical structure reminiscent of one's own backyard. Alternatively, it may serve as a metaphor for personal boundaries, limitations, protection, or separation. These interpretations, ranging from the concrete to the metaphysical, are all valid insofar as they reflect different worldviews and meaning-making processes.

Such interpretative openness is one reason photography has been successfully integrated within qualitative research paradigms. Qualitative inquiry typically aligns with an idealist

DOI: 10.4324/9781003537540-2

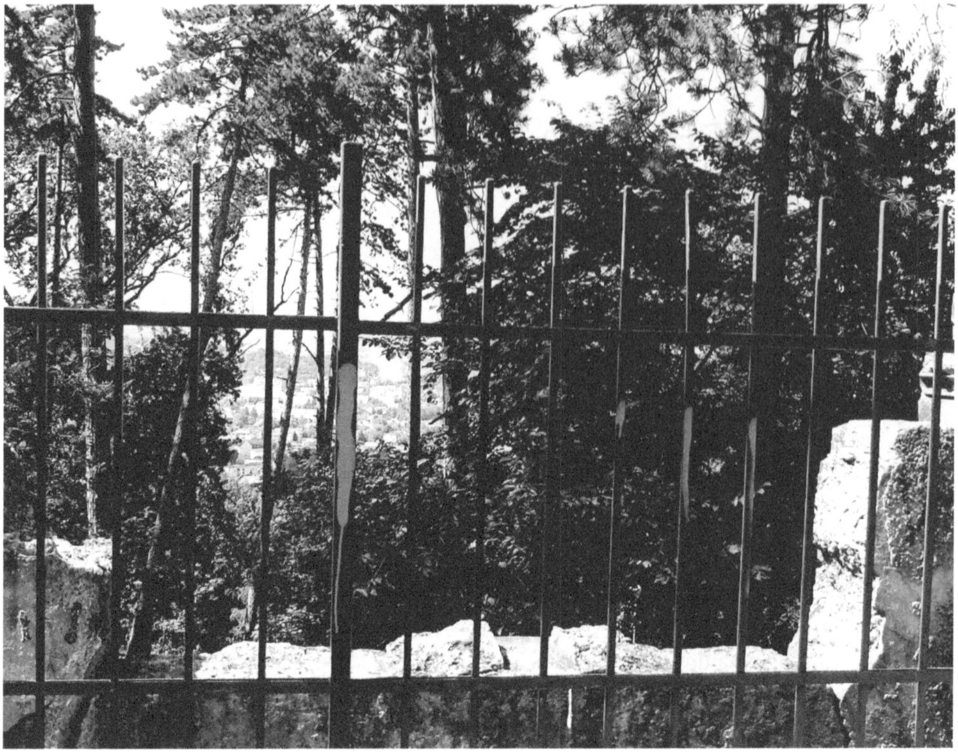

FIGURE 1.1 "There is freedom if you know how to see it. But you must go on the other side of the fence" (the fence as a symbol of the limitations imposed by living with a mental health condition)

Source: photograph and text by Rodion

ontological stance, which posits that reality can also be understood not only through material representations but also through the exploration of subjective experience, thought, and meaning. This perspective challenges the scientific-realist assumptions rooted in positivism that reality is solely material and can be fully captured through quantitative methods (Spencer et al., 2014).

Inevitably, this discussion extends to the role of photography in exploring human consciousness and the phenomenology of photography. Phenomenology has been critically examined within philosophy and across various other disciplines. For the purpose of this chapter, phenomenology is defined more broadly as "the study of structures of consciousness as experienced from the first-person point of view" (Smith, 2018, p. 1).

Health-related experiences such as stroke, post-natal depression, dental anxiety, and insomnia, to name only a few, serve as examples of phenomena that can be explored phenomenologically. To investigate such experiences, researchers may employ objective measurements and standardised assessments characteristic to quantitative research, often regarded as more empirical and scientific in nature. Alternatively, qualitative inquiry engages with individuals' perspectives, attitudes, behaviours, and meaning-making processes to access deeper understanding of lived experiences. This approach requires engagement with individuals' self-consciousness, which may be *pre-reflective* (primary or immediate) or *reflective* (second-order cognition) (Sartre, 1957).

For example, an individual may be aware of experiencing shortness of breath without actively contemplating it (pre-reflective consciousness). Upon being questioned by another individual who notices signs of discomfort, they may enter a reflective state, considering in greater depth how the experience feels, its underlying causes, and its broader implications (reflective consciousness). In this reflective process, individuals may articulate health-related anxieties or recognise the ways in which such symptoms impact on their quality of life and ability to engage in physical activities. In other words, reflective consciousness not only shapes individual perspectives on health experiences but also contributes to a richer understanding of the phenomenon for both the individual and others.

Photography can serve as a powerful tool for facilitating the transition from pre-reflective to reflective consciousness. In the same way that verbal prompts or interpersonal dialogue may invite an individual to reflect more deeply on their embodied experiences, photographs – whether taken by the individual or presented to them – can act as visual cues that elicit introspection and meaning-making. Through engagement with photographic images, individuals can externalise and re-encounter their experiences from a new perspective, facilitating not only self-reflection but also the articulation of thoughts and feelings that may otherwise remain unexpressed. In this way, photography becomes more than a representational tool; it becomes a reflective device that supports the transition from implicit, pre-reflective awareness to explicit, reflective understanding.

Some scholars refer to this potential as the "photographic phenomenology" (Pettersson, 2011). Phenomenology, as a philosophical approach, is primarily concerned with the study of the "appearance of things" – derived from the Greek *phainómenon* (that which appears) and *lógos* (study) – and focuses on how phenomena are subjectively experienced. In a similar way, photography can be seen as a medium that facilitates this process of "appearance", by visually revealing dimensions of experience that may otherwise remain subconscious or unarticulated.

While this is not the appropriate space for an in-depth exploration of the various phenomenological traditions, a basic distinction is necessary to clarify the theoretical underpinnings relevant to this discussion. Broadly, phenomenology can be divided into two primary strands: (1) *descriptive phenomenology*, which aims to understand phenomena as they are experiences in their raw form, free from the researcher's preconceptions and assumptions – a perspective rooted in the work of Edmund Husserl; and (2) *interpretive phenomenology*, which seeks to uncover meanings embedded within lived experience, understood in relation to the individual's socio-cultural and existential context. The latter approach, grounded in Heidegger's concept of *being-in-the-world*, aligns with hermeneutics, described by Lopez and Willis (2004) as "a process and method for bringing out and making manifest what is normally hidden in human experience" (p. 728).

This interpretive lens is essential for understanding the epistemological potential of photography as a research method. Beyond its anecdotal or documentary function, photography – when used as a *photo-instrument* – has the potential "to make visible what otherwise may remain hidden" (Sitvast, 2014, p. 18). In this sense, photographs as the one shown in Figure 1.2 do not merely depict objects or moments but also act as semiotic devices that invite deeper exploration of meaning, facilitate its construction, and enable its communication within research contexts.

A discussion of phenomenology within healthcare research would be incomplete without introducing the concept of embodiment. Embodiment, a core principle within phenomenological

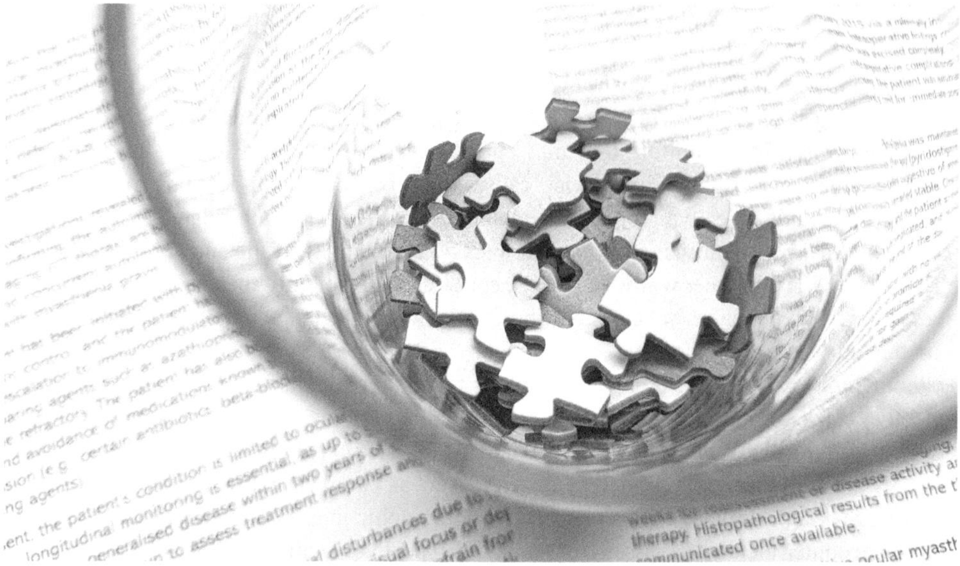

FIGURE 1.2 "Behind the diagnosis"

Source: photograph by the Author

philosophy, refers to the body's central role in shaping perception, experience, and engagement with the world (Fernandez, 2020). This concept is particularly relevant in understanding health and illness, as bodily experience is not a simple, passive reflection of disease but an active, dynamic process through which individuals interpret and respond to their conditions. The relationship between the body and health phenomena is thus inherently synergistic.

A key contribution to the philosophical framing of embodiment comes from Maurice Merleau-Ponty, a French philosopher who brought the *body* back on the pedestal of human experience after being separated or dualised from the *mind* by classical thinkers like Descartes. Merleau-Ponty (1962) argued that the body is not an object one possesses, but rather the very medium through which we experience the world. In his view, human existence is fundamentally embodied, and the body is inseparable from personal identity and perceptual experience. Essentially, Merleau-Ponty emphasises the phenomenological idea of *being-in-the-world* while living in a *body* that cannot exist separately from who we are, from our personal identity, and our perception of the surrounding world.

In psychological terms, this aspect was coined as *embodied cognition*, which posits that cognitive processes are influenced not only by the brain but also by the body's interaction with its surroundings (Goldman, 2012). Within photography, the implications of embodiment are two-fold: the body becomes both a subject that visually expresses meaning, and a medium through which lived experience is made visible. Moreover, the camera itself can be conceptualised as an extension of the body – a tactile, sensorial tool that externalises thought, emotion, and sensation. In this way, photography functions not only as a means of representation but also as an embodied act of meaning-making. I included a set of photographs below that represents my embodied experience of living with ocular myasthenia gravis. It reflects not only clinical

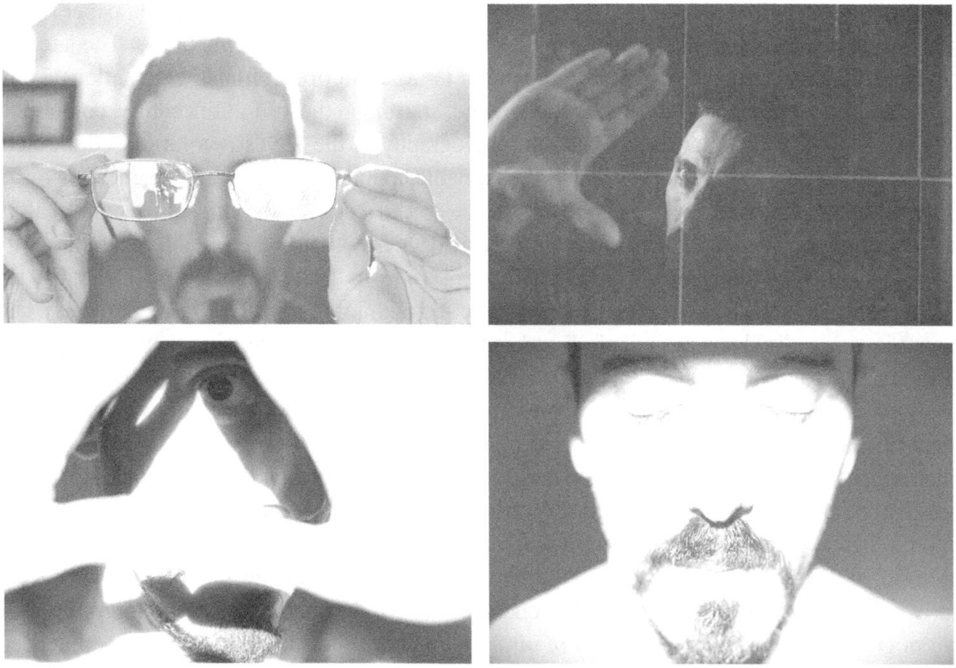

FIGURE 1.3 Photographic reflections on living with ocular myasthenia gravis

Source: photographs by the Author

symptoms such as ptosis (drooping eyelids) and diplopia (double vision) but also the deeper, lived reality that shapes how I perceive, identify, and interact with the world (Figure 1.3)

This section aimed to introduce the philosophical foundations for the use of photography as a method of knowledge generation within healthcare research. The alignment between photography and phenomenological philosophy emerges as particularly salient, owing to their shared emphasis on lived experience, perception, and meaning-making. As illustrated in this section, the conceptual parallels between photography and phenomenology provide an ideal framework for exploring the subjective dimensions of health and illness. Nonetheless, photography can be examined through numerous other philosophical lenses, both epistemically and aesthetically. While this chapter focuses primarily on phenomenological perspectives, additional readings are recommended at the end of the chapter for those interested in broader theoretical explorations such as critical realism, post-structuralism, post-modernism, semiotics, and visual hermeneutics.

1.2 A brief history of photography as a research method

The invention of photography by Nicéphore Niépce in the mid-1820s, followed by the development of the daguerreotype – a precursor to the modern photographic camera – by his associate Louis Daguerre, opened new technological horizons with potential to capture the world in unprecedented ways. This marked the beginning of a rapid progression from the metal photographic plates of the daguerreotype, which consisted of a sheet of copper plated with a thin cover of silver, to Talbot's paper-based process utilising calotype techniques, i.e., paper treated with silver iodide, which preceded the advent of glass-based photographic plates. The late 19th century witnessed another significant innovation in the form of roll films, which allowed photographers to capture black-and-white images and, starting in the mid-20th century, colour photographs. Finally, the emergence of digital photography in the 1990s revolutionised the field, making photography more accessible and sustainable, akin to contemporary practices.

The use of photography in healthcare can be traced back to the mid-nineteenth century, shortly after the introduction of the commercial daguerreotype. One notable example is the photographs of asylum patients in England from 1845 to 1920, analysed by Dahlquist and Kinderman (2023), who contextualised this practice within the transition in mental healthcare from viewing individuals as "lunatics" and "social outcasts" to recognising them as "patients". Although the camera in the asylums was not initially employed as a research method per se, the photographs of patients served to complement their medical records. In line with a positivist view of reality – objective, realistic, and representative of the scientific or empirical truth – photography was regarded by psychiatrists as an invaluable tool for understanding mental health conditions and their treatment. For instance, photographs were used to provide insights into biological pathologies and phenotypes, along with their progression, by capturing multiple portraits of the same patient throughout their journey through "madness". This is supported by early publications such as Hugh W. Diamond's (1857) *On the application of photography to the physiognomic and mental phenomena of insanity*, in which the author, Medical Superintendent of the Surrey Lunatic Asylum, highlights the functionality of "the portraits of the insane":

> It is well known that the portraits of those who are congregated in prisons for punishment have often time been of much value in recapturing some who have escaped, or improving with little expense, and with certainty a previous conviction and similarly the portraits of the Insane who are received into Asylums for protection, give to the eye so clear a representation of their case that on their re-admission after temporary absence and cure.
>
> *(Diamond, 1857, p. 7)*

Applications of photography in the 19th-century asylums exemplify an early form of *scientific photography* (Tucker, 2019), dedicated to capturing natural phenomena across various disciplines such as astronomy, chemistry, microbiology, and physics. Scientific and naturalistic investigations have consistently required the documentation of the world, particularly in its material form, through photographic production to consolidate the foundations of knowledge. Pierre Jules César Janssen (1877, in Hayden, 2008) asserted that photography was the "true retina of the scientist", capable of perceiving what the human eye cannot normally see. The integration of the daguerreotype with a microscope dates back to the 1840s, when Alfred François Donné photographed sections of bones and teeth at the Charité Hospital in Paris. This practice marked the beginning of medical photography, which has been frequently employed in neurology, dermatology, and dentistry, among other clinical areas, for diagnostic purposes and for documenting medical conditions throughout the stages of treatment.

The interpretivist perspective challenged the objective way of seeing the world through the viewfinder of the photographic camera, positing that it is not possible to attain objective knowledge of social realities through empirical means, as with the natural world (Gadamer, 2004). This argument is based on the premise that researchers are inherently part of the world they study, and thus, they possess a pre-understanding of social phenomena that inevitably influences their inquiry. Consequently, there are multiple, equally valid truths and ways to perceive the world. This perspective coincided with a shift in photography towards a more subjective approach. A notable international trend in this context is *subjective photography* (*Subjektive Fotografie*), founded by the German medical doctor and photographer Otto Steiner in the 1950s. Steiner moved away from the documentary and commercial "straight" use of photography towards a more experimental and artistic form, which is described as "humanised, individualised photography that implies the handling of a camera in order to win from the single object the views expressive of its character" (Steiner, 1954, pp. 26–27). Steiner's work revived the avant-garde photography of the 1920s and reinforced photography's status as a creative medium that encapsulates metaphysical representations of reality. Furthermore, photography became a vector of meanings open to interpretation. This era in photography intersected with Gadamer's philosophical work, which built on Heidegger's hermeneutics, centred around the idea of experience and reflection as pathways to discovering deeper understandings of reality (Greenwald, 1992).

One of the most iconic applications of photography as a research method in anthropology is exemplified by the monograph *Balinese character: A photographic analysis* by Bateson and Mead (1942). This work aimed to "translate aspects of culture . . . into some form of communication sufficiently clear and sufficiently unequivocal to satisfy the requirements of scientific enquiry", and to "communicate those intangible aspects of culture . . . in an attempt to describe the way in which the emotional life of these various South Sea peoples was organised in culturally standardised forms" (p. xi). The methodological rigour of the approach proposed by Bateson and Mead faced criticism at the time for being more journalistic than scientific, relying heavily on literary skill, and being difficult to replicate and evaluate. Coincidentally, some of the critiques of early research methods incorporating photography echoed the backlash against qualitative approaches promoted in the 1940s by Paul Felix Lazersfield (in Fleck, 2015). Despite this, anthropologists and sociologists continued to develop photographic methods, which found fertile ground in the methodology and philosophy of qualitative research.

A significant milestone in the evolution of visual ethnography is the introduction of photo-elicitation interviews by John Collier in the 1950s. Collier, an American anthropologist recognised as a methodological pioneer in this field, published the seminal article *Photography in anthropology: A report on two experiments* (Collier, 1957). This article, based on two research projects – one of which was an interdisciplinary study on the relationship between the environment and mental health – advocated for the potential of photography to "widen the field of scientific recognition and accelerate the processes of research" (p. 843). Collier emphasised the use of "photographs as an aid to interviewing" and the possibility of triangulating visual data with field notes. He challenged the traditional illustrative function of photography in anthropology, aiming to capture the subjective dimension of human experience: "We are not so much concerned with how a man looks as with what a man thinks" (p. 844).

Collier advanced the concept of the photograph as a "cultural map", guiding research participants towards insights pertinent to his project. He conducted comparative studies by dividing the interviewees into groups with and without photographs, concluding that "the photographic interview got considerably more concrete information on the structure and processes . . . more empathetic expressions . . . and much more specific information" compared to non-photographic interviews. Collier's narrative article reveals his enthusiasm for the emerging research method he termed *photo-elicitation*, in which "the imagery opened doors of memory and released emotions about forgotten circumstances . . . and triggered responses that might lie submerged in verbal interviewing" (p. 853–854).

Collier's work provides early insights into the comparative effectiveness of photo-elicitation interviews, which were "impressively longer and more complete than the non-picture interviews that were less structured, rambling, and freer in association" (p. 856–857). A decade later, Collier published his seminal work *Visual anthropology: Photography as a research method* (1967), recommended as further reading at the end of the chapter. Although not directly related to health research, Collier's book encapsulates over three decades of research experience, offering invaluable insights into the use of photography as a tool to explore human behaviour and culture. The significance of Collier's work is reflected in its wide range of applications across anthropology, sociology, psychology, and health sciences. The latter will be explored in more depth in Chapter 2.

Photo-elicitation involves the incorporation of photographs taken by the researcher, the research participant, or sourced from elsewhere, to elicit subjective information such as thoughts, feelings, attitudes, or to evoke narratives and memories, depending on research context. However, the use of photography soon transcended the confines of qualitative one-to-one interviewing, with photographs becoming instrumental in advocacy, activism, and social change. One of the most prominent applications of photography as a catalyst for community change is *photovoice*, a photographic technique developed in the late 1990s by Wang and Burris (1997). In essence, photovoice empowers participants by providing them with cameras to (1) document and reflect their community's strengths and concerns; (2) promote critical dialogue and knowledge about significant issues through group discussions of photographs; and (3) engage policymakers. Although photovoice is more prominent within social sciences, it originated in health promotion and has been extensively employed in various areas of health research discussed in the subsequent chapter. Notably, photovoice aligns with the emancipatory social developments in the 1980s and 1990s, driven by the global human rights and disability movements, feminism, and the pursuit of socio-economic justice, which called for advocacy tools in both society and research. Consequently, photovoice is frequently regarded as a form of participatory action research aimed at addressing social injustice and facilitating social change by those with first-hand experience of community issues (Falconer, 2014).

Photo-elicitation and photovoice are two pivotal techniques in the history of photography-based research, employed in various ways to meet the specific needs and objectives of a study. Regardless of their application, these techniques exemplify the use of photography as a tool for exploring human experiences that are challenging to investigate through non-photographic methods. The role of photography in journalism can be considered as an example. Without photographs, the social impact of storytelling, perception, and memory would be significantly diminished. Moreover, the credibility of a story could be compromised without photographic documentation. While the purpose of research differs from that of journalism, it similarly involves narrating the findings of social, economic, or health enquiries. Although images may not always be necessary, their inclusion undoubtedly enhances the depth of knowledge, leading to a more comprehensive understanding of the phenomena under investigation.

1.3 Rationale for employing photography in healthcare research

The application of photography in healthcare research has predominantly been clinical until recent years. Clinical photographers document various health conditions to provide supporting evidence for diagnosis and treatment. Examples include dermoscopic photography, which captures changes in moles or other skin conditions during treatment; pre-, intra-, and post-operative photography in plastic surgery; and medico-legal photography, which serves as evidence in lawsuits and claims.

The clinical use of photography is well-documented in research. For instance, Rogers et al. (2022) found that dermoscopic photographs increased the accuracy of malignancy recognition. Tabata et al. (2022) advocate for dental photography to enhance the communication between professionals and patients. Tang and Raju (2015) emphasise the importance of accurate photographic documentation in clinical endoscopy procedures as an integral aspect of quality control in endoscopic interventions. These advancements are facilitated by the widespread use of digital photography and mobile devices, which provide sharp, high-quality images. Consequently, objective medical photographs can complement textual information in health records and serve as a valuable educational resource for staff, students, and patients.

In recent years, photographs have been increasingly utilised in research in more innovative ways, extending beyond their traditional role of accurately depicting physical manifestations of health and illness. This shift may be attributed to the non-material or experiential aspects of physical and mental health that cannot be clinically captured. Consider the example of lived experience, which encompasses first-hand knowledge from individuals living with a health condition, along with its social, psychological, and cultural complexities. In research, health experiences are often conveyed through narrative storytelling, where individuals share their perspectives and understanding of a health issue. Parker et al. (2024) offer an insightful exploration of living with and managing the invisible symptoms of multiple sclerosis using photovoice. This methodology enabled the authors to enrich the collected data, leading to a more nuanced understanding of how the research participants manage their symptoms and interpret the meaning attached to their lived experience. This perspective is echoed in one of my phenomenological studies which employs photographic techniques to elicit participant discussions around the meanings and experiences of mental health recovery (Milasan, 2024).

Although these examples originate from various subject areas, they collectively demonstrate the benefits of using images to enhance research and provide qualitative inquiry with an additional layer of depth. Cleland and MacLeod (2021) advocate for visual methodologies to challenge the "linguistic imperialism" of textual data. Their perspective is widely supported by literature that employs photography as a source of participant data, asserting that photo-elicitation interviews, for instance, can yield insights that are otherwise impossible to capture through traditional text-based interviews. A plausible explanation for the advantages of photography-based data collection tools, compared with non-photographic methods, can be found in evolutionary studies of brain development (Harper, 2002). It is well-established that areas of the human brain responsible for processing visual cues are older than those associated with verbal information. Consequently, photography facilitates (re)surfacing of information from the depths of consciousness and elevates our understanding of experiences by enabling access to thoughts and feelings that are difficult to articulate verbally (Harper, 2002). Although these conclusions initially emerged from sociological and anthropological research, they are equally applicable to healthcare-related subjects investigated through photographic methods. This was evident in one of my studies exemplified above (Milasan, 2024), where I realised that I could not have fully comprehended the cultural and environmental contexts of mental health recovery without the aid of the photographs.

Based on this premise, I advocated for the use of photography as a tool for situating the subject under investigation within the lifeworld of participants, as they explore it through the viewfinder of the camera, in a literature review on this topic (Milasan et al., 2022). Consider, for instance, the challenges of exploring a sensitive topic like mental health in a traditional interview, where participants would be expected to convey information solely through words. When addressing the environment and culture in which such experiences occur, the difficulty increases, as participants may be so immersed in their own worlds that they take socio-cultural aspects for granted and may omit them from their narratives.

Photography mitigates this limitation by allowing researchers to gain a literal glimpse into participants' environments, which is often crucial for understanding their experiences. Through photography, descriptions become richer, resulting in a more comprehensive understanding of the phenomena under investigation. Consequently, the quality, trustworthiness, and credibility of the research can be potentially enhanced through photography by triangulating or corroborating visual and textual datasets (Hatzikiriakidis, 2023).

Based on the evidence presented so far, it may be inferred that the use of photography-based methods benefits researchers exclusively. However, the advantages of employing photographic techniques extend to research participants as well. For this reason, the use of photography in research is appealing from an ethical standpoint, when fundamental ethical principles such as beneficence or maximising the benefits for the research participants are considered, as outlined in the Belmont Report (Cassell, 2000). Researchers strive to ensure that there is a clear benefit for the research participants and other indirect beneficiaries from the activities, knowledge, and understanding generated throughout the research. Similarly, researchers adhere to the principle of non-maleficence, which entails minimising potential harm to research participants. Photography is known to provide an emotional buffer for participants while they explore potentially distressful experiences of health and illness (Milasan et al., 2022). As a result, photography becomes central to the research process, diverting participants' attention and allowing them to maintain emotional detachment. For instance, photographic metaphors, which will be discussed in greater detail in subsequent chapters, offer explorative opportunities beyond concrete realities that research participants may find difficult to articulate verbally.

Photography has the potential to enable the voices of research participants whose verbal abilities may be limited, such as individuals with learning disabilities, cerebral palsy, selective mutism, dementia or Alzheimer's, and other categories of non-verbal or minimally verbal individuals requiring alternative forms of communication. Photography has been increasingly used in exploring such experiences, contributing to enhanced inclusivity and participation in research, which might otherwise be constrained by data collection methods requiring high levels of cognitive engagement (Sigstad & Garrels, 2021). Therefore, it is not surprising that photography is embedded in participatory research due to its potential for collaboration and empowerment, echoing the ethical principle of autonomy.

Photography creates valuable opportunities for the research participants to engage in the decision-making process, such as the selection of photographs and photographic subjects, interpretation and analysis, and research dissemination. Moreover, photography helps to minimise the power imbalance between researchers and participants by providing a research tool over which the participants have greater control and freedom (Milasan et al., 2022). This process results in a shift from the dominant discourse of health professionals and researchers to those with first-hand experience of health who take ownership of their photographs and narratives, and portray them in ways they consider relevant and appropriate. Ethically, this aspect aligns with the principle of justice and equitable representation in research.

Occupational aspects of health and illness have been extensively evidenced in the literature, demonstrating the benefits of meaningful occupations for the recovery of individuals experiencing various physical and/or mental health conditions that profoundly disrupt their lives and levels of functioning. Photography, for instance, has been identified as a significant form of occupational therapy, contributing to the development of practical and cognitive abilities and fostering personal and social transformation in individuals living with mental health difficulties (Kearns-Murphy & Fox, 2024) and developmental disabilities (Edrisinha et al., 2011). However, the therapeutic benefits of photography as a research method extend beyond occupational aspects. The next section looks more closely at the therapeutic value of photography, further supporting the rationale for employing photographic techniques in health research.

1.4 The therapeutic value of photography as a research method

The integration of photography in health research is facilitated by its development as a therapeutic tool capitalising on its cathartic effects and its potential to reveal subconscious aspects of human experience. Photography opens avenues for expressing thoughts and emotions that verbal communication alone may not be able to convey. Consequently, its use in therapeutic environments has increased to enhance communication (Gibson, 2017). In their literature review, Saita and Tramontano (2018) identified various contexts in which photography is employed therapeutically: health and clinical settings, such as individuals diagnosed with chronic illnesses experiencing functional impairments like neurological diseases and cancers; social and community settings, including marginalised individuals at risk of social exclusion; and educational institutions, such as nursing students and recovery colleges. The widespread application of photography as a therapeutic approach may reflect a holistic and person-centred paradigm in healthcare, where the subjective dimensions of health experiences gain prominence alongside clinical aspects.

Photo-therapy (Weiser, 1999) and therapeutic photography (Loewenthal, 2013) are two established practices that utilise photographs for therapeutic purposes. While they share certain similarities, photo-therapy typically requires a trained counsellor or therapist, whereas therapeutic photography can be initiated independently by individuals or groups through more autonomous photo-based activities (Gibson, 2018). Despite their different methodologies, both practices emphasise the processual nature of taking photographs and their cathartic effects, rather than focusing solely on the photographs as creative outcomes. This process is crucial for understanding the therapeutic value of photography in health research, encompassing various steps such as taking pictures, selecting them, discussing and analysing, processing and post-processing through digital manipulation and collages, printing and disseminating them in different formats. This process actively engages research participants not only occupationally and recreationally but also therapeutically, although the primary aim of research may differ from therapy focused on psychological healing. Nevertheless, embedding photography in research can create opportunities to explore its therapeutic value, thereby enhancing the benefits for research participants in line with the ethical principle of beneficence, as discussed in the previous section and elaborated upon in one of my articles (Milasan, 2024).

The literature indicates that the therapeutic value of photography is deeply intertwined with self and identity (Dollinger & Clancy, 1993). Portraiture, self-portraiture, and the contemporary practice of taking selfies can reflect an individual's identity, revealing personal experiences, meanings, and social contexts, including ethnicity, gender, power dynamics, culture, family, and class. An informal discussion of a portrait can uncover a myriad of aspects for both the viewer and the subject of the photograph. Photography becomes, therefore, a tool or mediator for self-discovery and a powerful expression of identity with all its psycho-social complexities. As a result, a photo-elicitation interview may transcend a mere data collection encounter to address a research question; it may also provide an opportunity for self-discovery or even a revelation for participants, who may gain a deeper understanding of their health condition. This conclusion is supported by a literature review on the therapeutic benefits of participatory photography (Buchan, 2020). In this study, adults with mental health issues were found to engage in deep reflections on life, which positively impacted their recovery by helping them make sense of suffering and healing, and reframe their narratives from vulnerability to strength. Additionally, Buchan (2020) asserts that photographs also facilitated the development of therapeutic relationships between participants and professionals or the research team through enhanced communication and empowerment.

In a study I conducted with individuals experiencing mental health difficulties (Milasan, 2023), I had the privilege of witnessing the therapeutic value of photography-based research methods. Initially, I employed photography as an elicitation tool to enrich the qualitative data. However, shortly after initiating the research, I realised that photography was much more than a data collection tool for exploring participants' experiences of recovery; it emerged as a meaningful instrument for facilitating and supporting their recovery. In a reflective piece (Milasan, 2024), I elaborated on the insights gained from my study, which revolved around four key themes: photography as a means of forging social companionship and camaraderie, facilitating self-awareness and intra and interpersonal reflection, supporting meaningful connections with the natural environment, and serving as a therapeutic occupation.

Given the numerous therapeutic benefits of photography for research participants, it is unsurprising that it has been increasingly used in health research and other disciplines. The exponential growth of photography-based studies can be attributed not only to recent advancements in digital technology and the ease of accessing photographic tools but also to the inherent therapeutic value of these methods, which likely contributes to their appeal amongst research participants.

1.5 Limitations and challenges of photography-based research in healthcare

Photography-based techniques in health research, while appealing to both researchers and research participants, necessitate careful reflection and consideration. This is due to the numerous implications that may hinder or even compromise the process of designing and conducting photographic research. Despite the limitations and challenges being less frequently reported in the literature, a closer examination of studies employing photography at various stages of the research process reveals a multitude of issues that warrant attention.

Although photography as a method of data collection may initially be perceived as enjoyable and recreational by research participants, they may experience inhibition when it comes to sharing personal experiences of health and illness. This is particularly evident in group settings, where participants may fear being judged or looked down upon by their peers or researchers who may not relate to their experiences or perceive them negatively (Maniam et al., 2016).

Such experiences can adversely affect the emotional well-being of participants, particularly when they feel stuck and unable to complete their photographic missions. Additionally, the technical or artistic focus of photography can divert attention from the primary objectives of the project. For instance, a participant in one of my studies disclosed that taking photographs often triggered his perfectionism, leading to negative emotions such as anxiety, self-doubt, a reinforced sense of failure, and frustration. This was due to his perceived inability to capture the images he envisioned or the discrepancy between his ideal outcome and the final product of his photographic endeavours, which consistently disappointed him. Consequently, the participant chose to continue the study without taking photographs, providing an opportunity to explore this issue in greater depth. As someone passionate about photography and fully converted to the benefits of photographic research, this was both a challenging experience and a revelation, prompting me to reflect more deeply on the unintended negative impacts of using photography on research participants.

Group settings, such as photography workshops, may be limited in facilitating the disclosure of personal experiences and aspects perceived as socially undesirable, like self-harm, suicidal thoughts, overdosing, non-adherence to prescribed treatments, or negative lifestyles. Therefore, some participants may prefer one-to-one photo-elicitation interviews, where peer pressure is not a concern, although this does not guarantee greater comfort in disclosing such issues. For this reason, it is recommended that research participants are adequately informed about the nature of the photographic activities and given the option to participate in either groups or one-to-one activities. This approach may also positively impact the ethical aspects of the research, including considerations of participants' needs and preferences.

Another aspect of photography-based research that may induce anxiety in participants is the technical difficulties they may encounter while using photographic equipment. I have worked with individuals who had not previously taken digital photographs, which may be a common occurrence in certain cultural and social contexts, such as under-developed countries. Therefore, handling the camera was initially a stressful experience for some, including the fear of damaging the equipment.

Additionally, the technical language of photography can be intimidating. Participants may also experience feelings of embarrassment, particularly when there are tech-savvy individuals in photography groups. To address this, I tend to capitalise on the diverse digital skills within photography groups to facilitate mutual support and mentoring, which positively impacts group dynamics and atmosphere. Alternatively, incorporating more preparatory sessions to help participants build confidence in using the equipment should be factored in the research schedule.

Photography can indeed be an uncertain emotional terrain, where its therapeutic value may be unexpectedly replaced with adverse effects impacting the psychological well-being of research participants. Photographs can serve as an emotional buffer, diverting attention from personal experiences to the object of photography or photographic metaphors that act as vectors for expressing thoughts and emotions (Switzer, 2019). However, photography can also evoke feelings and thoughts that may be psychologically harmful to participants. Therefore, it is imperative to carefully consider debriefing opportunities in photography-based health research, facilitated by trained psychologists, therapists, or counsellors.

Using photography in research can also raise safety concerns, particularly in marginalised communities where photography may be perceived as being intrusive or even offensive. Open discussions with research participants and informing them about ethical considerations surrounding photography at the onset of the project can help address such issues. This may involve obtaining consent for taking pictures of other individuals or agreeing not to photograph others altogether, depending on the research topic. I have often had to negotiate this aspect with participants who took photographs of others without permission, despite being provided with instructions and consent forms. Ethical implications may be exacerbated in deprived communities where carrying an expensive camera or photographing individuals who may be gang members or drug dealers, as noted in Padgett et al.'s (2013) study, could result in unintended harm to research participants. This does not imply that participants should be provided with disposable cameras. While inexpensive equipment has been widely used in research for cost-effectiveness, it may negatively impact the sense of worth of research participants (Milasan, 2023).

Additional ethical considerations related to photographic research in healthcare are discussed in detail in Chapter 7. A key takeaway from this section is the ethical responsibility and accountability of researchers utilising photography to remain alert to any inadvertent physical and psychological implications of employing photographic techniques in their studies. Given that research participants may already be in vulnerable social, psychological, and physical positions, it is imperative to avoid causing further distress or complications to their circumstances. Therefore, it is essential to provide participants with the opportunity to reflect on, and verbalise, the limitations and challenges they experience when using photography at all stages of a research project.

Conclusion

Photography has evolved from a technical innovation into a profound epistemological and methodological resource for healthcare research. Its unique ability to bridge material and experiential dimensions of health makes it more than a tool for documentation – it becomes a medium for meaning-making, reflection, and empowerment. By aligning with phenomenological principles, photography enables researchers to access lived experiences that often remain hidden behind clinical narratives, while offering participants opportunities for self-expression and identity work. At the same time, its therapeutic potential reinforces ethical commitments to beneficence and inclusivity, positioning photography as both a research instrument and a catalyst for well-being. Yet, this promise is tempered by emotional, technical, and ethical challenges that demand careful consideration. As healthcare research continues to embrace visual methodologies, photography invites us to rethink what counts as evidence, how knowledge is constructed, and how research can remain responsive to the complexities of human experience.

Knowledge check

1. What do photography and phenomenology have in common from a philosophical perspective?
2. What are the milestones of photography-based research from a historical perspective?
3. Why can photography be a valuable research method for researchers and research participants?
4. What does the therapeutic value of photography-based research consist of?
5. Identify five challenges to using photography in healthcare research and reflect on their implications for researchers and research participants.

References

Barthes, R. (1993). *Camera Lucida* (R. Howard, Trans.). Vintage Classics.

Bateson, G., & Mead, M. (1942). *Balinese character. A photographic analysis*. New York Academy of Sciences

Buchan, C. A. (2020). Therapeutic benefits and limitations of participatory photography for adults with mental health problems: A systematic search and literature review. *Journal of Psychiatric and Mental Health Nursing, 27*(1), 657–668. https://doi.org/10.1111/jpm.12606

Cassell, E. J. (2000). The principles of the Belmont report revisited. How have respect for persons, beneficence, and justice been applied to clinical medicine? *Hastings Center Report, 30*(4), 12–21. https://doi.org/10.2307/3527640
Cleland, J., & MacLeod, A. (2021). The visual vernacular: Embracing photographs in research. *Perspectives on Medical Education, 10*(4), 230–237. https://doi.org/10.1007/S40037-021-00672-X
Collier, J. (1957). Photography in anthropology: A report on two experiments. *American Anthropologist, 59*(1), 843–859. https://www.jstor.org/stable/665849
Dahlquist, C., & Kinderman, P. (2023). 'Picture imperfect': The motives and uses of patient photography in the asylum. *History of Psychiatry, 34*(2), 130–145. https://doi.org/10.1177/0957154X231157001
Diamond, H. W. (1857). On the application of photography to the physiognomic and mental phenomena of insanity. *Proceedings of the Royal Society of London*. https://doi.org/10.1098/rspl.1856.0036
Dollinger, S. J., & Clancy, S. M. (1993). Identity, self, and personality: II. Glimpses through the autophotographic eye. *Journal of Personality and Social Psychology, 64*(6), 1064–1071. https://doi.org/10.1037/0022-3514.64.6.1064
Edrisinha, C., O'Reilly, M. F., Choi, H. Y., Sigafoos, J., & Lancioni, G. E. (2011). "Say cheese": Teaching photography skills to adults with developmental disabilities. *Research in Developmental Disabilities, 32*(2), 636–642. https://doi.org/10.1016/j.ridd.2010.12.006
Falconer, J. (2014). Photovoice participatory-action research design and adaptations for adverse fieldwork conditions. In *Sage research methods cases (part 1)*. SAGE Publications Ltd.
Fernandez, A. V. (2020). Embodiment and objectification in illness and health care: Taking phenomenology from theory to practice. *Journal of Clinical Nursing, 29*(21-22), 4403–4412. https://doi.org/10.1111/jocn.15431
Fleck, C. (2015). *Lazarsfeld, Paul Felix (1901–76)*. Elsevier.
Gadamer, H. G. (2004). *Truth and method*. Continuum.
Gibson, N. (2017). Therapeutic photography: Enhancing patient communication. *Journal of Kidney Care, 2*(1), 46–47. https://doi.org/10.12968/jokc.2017.2.1.46
Gibson, N. (2018). *Therapeutic photography: Enhancing self-esteem, self-efficacy and resilience*. Jessica Kingsley Publishers.
Goldman, A. I. (2012). A moderate approach to embodied cognitive science. *Review of Philosophy and Psychology, 3*(1), 71–88. https://doi.org/10.1007/s13164-012-0089-0
Greenwald, C. (1992). Photography as art in Heidegger's philosophy. *Episteme, 3*(1), Article 3. https://digitalcommons.denison.edu/episteme/vol3/iss1/3
Harper, D. (2002). Talking about pictures: A case for photo elicitation. *Visual Studies, 17*(1), 13–26. https://doi.org/10.1080/14725860220137345
Hatzikiriakidis, K. (2023). Photovoice. In D. Ayton, T. Tsindos, & D. Berkovic (Eds.), *Qualitative Research – a practical guide for health and social care researchers and practitioners*. Monash University.
Hayden, E. (2008). A snapshot of hidden science history. *Nature, 455*, 1180. https://doi.org/10.1038/4551180a
Kearns-Murphy, C., & Fox, J. (2024). Turning on "the Photographer mind": Experiences of mental health service users in a tutor-led photography group in an Irish context. *Occupational Therapy in Mental Health, 41*(2), 157–177. https://doi.org/10.1080/0164212X.2024.2340564
Loewenthal, D. (2013). *Phototherapy and therapeutic photography in a digital age* (1st ed.). Routledge.
Lopez, K. A., & Willis, D. G. (2004). Descriptive versus interpretive phenomenology: Their contributions to nursing knowledge. *Qualitative Health Research, 14*(5), 726–735. https://doi.org/10.1177/1049732304263638
Maniam, Y., Kumaran, P., Lee, Y. P., Koh, J., & Subramaniam, M. (2016). The journey of young people in an early psychosis program involved in participatory photography. *British Journal of Occupational Therapy, 79*(6), 368–375. https://doi.org/10.1177/0308022615621567
Merleau-Ponty, M. (1962). *Phenomenology of perception*. Routledge.
Milasan, L. H. (2023). "Mending fractured personalities": A photography-based cultural study of recovery from mental distress in Romania. *Transcultural Psychiatry, 60*(2), 226–243. https://doi.org/10.1177/13634615221119373
Milasan, L. H. (2024). 'Taking pictures is like treasure hunting': Exploring the therapeutic value of photography as a qualitative research method. *International Journal of Qualitative Methods, 23*(1), 1–20. https://doi.org/10.1177/16094069241236219
Milasan, L. H., Bingley, A. F., & Fisher, N. R. (2022). The big picture of recovery: A systematic review on the evidence of photography-based methods in researching recovery from mental distress. *Arts Health, 14*(2), 165–185. https://doi.org/10.1080/17533015.2020.1855453

Padgett, D. K., Smith, B. T., Derejko, K.-S., Henwood, B. F., & Tiderington, E. (2013). A picture is worth . . .? Photo elicitation interviewing with formerly homeless adults. *Qualitative Health Research, 23*(11), 1435–1444. https://doi.org/10.1177/1049732313507752

Parker, L.-S., Topcu, G., De Boos, D., Bale, C., & das Nair, R. (2024). Seeing the invisible: A photovoice exploration of living with and managing the invisible symptoms of multiple sclerosis. *Clinical Psychological Science, 12*(6), 1127–1145. https://doi.org/10.1177/21677026231220846

Pettersson, M. (2011). Depictive traces: On the phenomenology of photography. *Journal of Aesthetics and Art Criticism, 69*(2), 185–196. http://www.jstor.org/stable/42635475

Rogers, T., McCrary, M. R., Yeung, H., Krueger, L., & Chen, S. C. (2022). Dermoscopic photographs impact confidence and management of remotely triaged skin lesions. *Dermatology Practical & Conceptual, 12*(3), e2022129. https://doi.org/10.5826/dpc.1203a129

Saita, E., & Tramontano, M. (2018). Navigating the complexity of the therapeutic and clinical use of photography in psychosocial settings: A review of the literature. *Research in Psychotherapy, 21*(1), 293. https://doi.org/10.4081/ripppo.2018.293

Sartre, J.-P. (1957). *The transcendence of the ego: An existentialist theory of consciousness*. Octagon Books.

Sigstad, H. M. H., & Garrels, V. (2021). A semi-structured approach to photo elicitation methodology for research participants with intellectual disability. *International Journal of Qualitative Methods, 20*(1), 1–10. https://doi.org/10.1177/16094069211027057

Sitvast, J. (2014). Hermeneutic photography: An innovative intervention in psychiatric rehabilitation founded on concepts from Ricoeur. *Journal of Psychiatric Nursing, 5*(1), 17–24. https://doi.org/10.5505/phd.2014.69772

Smith, D. W. (2018). Phenomenology. In E. N. Zalta (Ed.), *The Stanford encyclopedia of philosophy*. Stanford University. https://plato.stanford.edu/archives/sum2018/entries/phenomenology

Spencer, R., Pryce, J. M., & Walsh, J. (2014). 5 philosophical approaches to qualitative research. In *Oxford handbook of qualitative research* (pp. 81–98). https://doi.org/10.1093/oxfordhb/9780199811755.013.027

Steiner, O. (1954). *Subjektive Fotografie*. State School of Arts.

Switzer, S. (2019). Working with photo installation and metaphor: Re-visioning photovoice research. *International Journal of Qualitative Methods, 18*(1), 1–14. https://doi.org/10.1177/1609406919872395

Tabata, L., Arcuri, T., & Hilgert, L. (2022). Dental photography as a key to clinical success. In D. Oliveira (Ed.), *Color science and shade selection in operative dentistry* (pp. 53–73). Springer.

Tang, S.-J., & Raju, G. (2015). Endoscopic photography and image documentation. *Gastrointestinal Endoscopy, 82*(5), 925–931. https://doi.org/10.1016/j.gie.2015.05.050

Tucker, J. (2019). Photography and the making of modern science. In G. Pasternak (Ed.), *The handbook of photography studies*. Routledge.

Wang, C., & Burris, M. A. (1997). Photovoice: Concept, methodology, and use for participatory needs assessment. *Health Education & Behavior, 24*(3), 369–387. https://doi.org/10.1177/109019819702400309

Weiser, J. (1999). *Phototherapy techniques: Exploring the secrets of personal snapshots and family albums* (2nd ed.). PhotoTherapy Centre.

Further reading

Cohen, J., & Meskin, A. (2004). On the epistemic value of photographs. *The Journal of Aesthetics and Art Criticism, 62*(2), 197–210. https://doi.org/10.1111/j.1540-594X.2004.00152.x

Collier, J. (1967). *Visual anthropology: Photography as a research method*. University of New Mexico Press.

Costello, D., & Phillips, D. M. (2009). Automatism, causality and realism: Foundational problems in the philosophy of photography. *Philosophy Compass, 4*(1), 1–21. https://doi.org/10.1111/j.1747-9991.2008.00193.x

Maynard, P. (1997). *The engine of visualization: Thinking through photography*. Cornell University Press.

2

PHOTOGRAPHIC APPROACHES TO HEALTHCARE RESEARCH

2.1 Photo-elicitation

In the previous chapter, photo-elicitation was introduced as a prominent form of photographic research, with its applications in sociology and anthropology dating back from the 1950s when John Collier pioneered this concept (Collier, 1957, 1967). Since its inception, photo-elicitation has been adapted to various areas of research, yet it fundamentally remains "a technique that incorporates photographs into research interviews, allowing for reflexivity between image and verbalisation to produce data" (Kyololo et al., 2023, p. 1). Although most studies refer to this method as *photo-elicitation*, the terminology may vary, including terms such as *photo-feedback*, *photo-interviewing*, *autodriving interviews*, and *reflexive photography* (Soaita & McKee, 2020). Some scholars (Hurworth et al., 2005) consider photovoice a subset of photo-elicitation. However, in this chapter, photo-elicitation and photovoice are examined as distinct techniques despite their common roots. This distinction is based on the differing participatory levels and other particularities that must be considered when selecting the most appropriate photography-based method.

The efficacy of photo-elicitation approaches in health research can be attributed to the potential of images to enhance the interview experience and add depth to qualitative data (Harper, 2002). This was illustrated in the first wave of photo-elicitation studies within the health domain during the 1990s and early 2000s. Notable amongst these are the studies by Bender and Castro (2000) and Bender et al. (2001), which investigated prenatal care among immigrant Latina women, with a focus on perceptions of resilience and risk factors, and quality of prenatal care within this population. Although the authors interchangeably use the term *photo-elicitation* with *photo-narratives* or *qualitative interviews with photographic prompts*, they offer invaluable insights into the methodological use of photographs. Interestingly, in Bender et al.'s (2001) study, the photographs were taken by the research team, with assistance from staff at the prenatal clinics where the research was conducted, and subsequently used as prompts in interviews with the participants.

DOI: 10.4324/9781003537540-3

Although less common than participant-led photography, the use of photographs not taken by research participants is not unusual in photo-elicitation. This is exemplified in Sitvast's (2015) study on recovery in mental healthcare, which aimed to uncover the strengths that instilled hope and meaning in life in hospitalised patients with severe mental health conditions in the Netherlands. For this purpose, fifteen service users, who actively participated in the process, were photographed by a professional photographer over two years, with their consent. They were involved in decision-making regarding the set-up of photoshoots and the selection of photographs, in line with the action-based research framework guiding this study. Another distinctive feature of Sitvast's (2015) study was the involvement of staff, specifically mental health nurses, in the production of photographic materials as "mentors" or "travelling companions" on participants' journey to recovery. This approach led to an enhanced "sense of reciprocity and equivalence between service users and professionals" (Sitvast, 2015, p. 141), positively impacting the therapeutic relationship. In the "How It Has Been Done" section, Sitvast (2015) provided a blueprint for co-creating approaches to photo-elicitation. Less participatory in nature but equally insightful, Larivière et al.'s (2015) approach to photo-eliciting life stories of women with borderline personality disorder utilised pictures cut by participants from magazines to represent their experiences. Similarly, Greco et al. (2016) combined participant-generated photographs with images from the Internet to explore experiences of children with behavioural disorders in a Canadian school-based psychiatric setting.

The abundance of photo-elicitation studies in mental healthcare is not coincidental. A systematic review I conducted on this topic (Milasan et al., 2022) concluded that photography as a research method in mental health holds significant therapeutic value, as discussed in the previous chapter. However, the application of photo-elicitation is not limited to mental health care. On the contrary, a plethora of examples from both clinical and non-clinical health research underscore the flexibility and versatility of this method, adaptable to various contexts.

For example, Bukhave et al. (2015) investigated perspectives on participation in everyday occupations amongst individuals with hand osteoarthritis through participant-led photographs. The authors argue that photo-elicitation techniques were more engaging and reflexive compared to conventional interviews, particularly in capturing the embodied lived experiences of the research participants. In a more sensitive context, Rivard et al. (2022) employed photography to reveal deep emotions, memories, and perspectives on the post-treatment experiences of twenty rectal cancer survivors. Rivard et al. (2022) contended that allowing participants to provide their own images and discuss them in a more unstructured manner was beneficial when interviews involved delicate topics. Otherwise, such topics may trigger embarrassment and reluctance to take part in research: "the photographs help to overcome barriers and facilitate conversation, providing nuanced information on the illness experience while also providing anonymity and distance from sensitive issues" (Rivard et al., 2022, p. 2).

Photo-elicitation is frequently employed to explore experiences of health and illness in populations where language barriers may hinder the research process. For instance, Alsubhi et al. (2022) investigated the health behaviours of young children from refugee families relocated to the UK using participant-driven photo-elicitation techniques. This method provided "a viable, accessible way for participants to express and explain their experiences" (Alsubhi et al., 2022, p. 1104). Photo-elicitation is an optimal research method in healthcare studies involving children, who may struggle to articulate their thoughts and feelings. Additionally, children may feel intimidated by the researcher's presence, which introduces inherent power dynamics that can negatively impact the research process. Photography has increasingly been used to democratise research with young people, who have often been excluded on the basis that they may be less experienced and competent compared to adults. However, health studies integrating auto-driven photo-elicitation like Epstein et al.'s (2006) exploration of children with cancer's perspectives on, and responses to, a specialised summer camp, suggest otherwise. Similarly, photo-elicitation methods have successfully guided studies with people with dementia (Lood et al., 2023) and their carers (Rayment et al., 2019), underscoring its potential to facilitate older persons' participation in research.

As illustrated in the examples above, photo-elicitation is a versatile and diverse technique, allowing for creativity in the incorporation of photographs from various sources into the research process. However, this versatility leads to methodological inconsistencies, which may account for the gap in the literature regarding a standardised framework for conducting photo-elicitation research.

Drawing on my experience as a visual researcher and the literature reviewed on this topic, I have devised a step-by-step approach (Table 2.1) that can be tailored to the specific needs and particularities of various healthcare research contexts. Key steps, such as addressing ethical considerations, methods for data collection and analysis, will be elaborated upon in subsequent chapters, along with discussions on challenges and limitations, and potential solutions.

TABLE 2.1 Conducting a photo-elicitation study step-by-step (adapted from Milasan, 2022)

Step 1	Research participants are provided with cameras and instructed on their use; ethical considerations related to photography, as well as health and safety issues, are explained to participants.
Step 2	The researcher ensures that participants understand the research topic they are invited to represent visually, for example, through "photo-missions" negotiated with research participants.
Step 3	Participants capture images that represent the research topic and their experiences, typically within familiar environments or communities, over a certain period (e.g., one or two weeks prior to the interview).
Step 4	Participants, in collaboration with the researcher, select photographs. The researcher may recommend a limited number of photos per session to avoid repetition, ensure depth of data, represent the topic comprehensively, and also for time management purposes.
Step 5	Selected images are critically reflected upon in photo-elicitation interviews with a recommended duration of 30–90 minutes, photography workshops or focus groups lasting up to 2 hours, or a combination of these approaches.
	Photo-elicitation group activities, known to enhance social construction and negotiation of meanings, are typically facilitated by researchers and ideally involve 6–8 participants.
Step 6	Participants' interpretations of images inform data analysis, allowing the researcher to remain closely with the meanings attributed by informants to their photographic work.
Step 7	The researcher may label and organise photographs through tabulation and visual maps, or utilise specialised qualitative software (e.g., Atlas.ti®, NVivo®) to facilitate coding and thematic processing of visual material corroborated with textual data.
Step 8	Member-checking groups can be organised to create opportunities for participants to reflect on and provide feedback on preliminary or final findings, addressing any misunderstandings or misinterpretations that could impact on the methodological rigour of the study.

2.2 Photovoice

Photovoice is an influential photographic research method, briefly introduced in Chapter 1. Originally conceptualised by Caroline Wang and Mary Ann Burris in the 1990s, photovoice – initially termed *photo novella* – emerged from a pioneering study aimed at articulating the health needs of women from a Chinese community and conveying these to policymakers (Wang & Burris, 1994). Photovoice is rooted in the emancipatory principles of Freirean critical pedagogy (Freire, 1970), which emphasise education as a means of developing critical awareness of power dynamics in society.

Designed as an educational and participatory tool, photovoice seeks to empower marginalised populations by enabling them to challenge and transform oppressive social structures. The primary objective of photovoice, as envisaged by Wang and Burris (1994), is to amplify the voices of those often excluded from policy discourse by promoting dialogue, stimulating collective reflection, and catalysing social action. This approach seeks not only to generate knowledge but also to disseminate it in ways that inform policy and instigate community-driven change. As such, photovoice transcends the more conventional aims of photo-elicitation, which typically centres on data collection and interpretation. Instead, photovoice aligns with the principles of participatory action research (Wang, 1999), positioning participants as co-researchers actively engaged in both the identification of issues and the pursuit of transformative outcomes.

Photovoice has gained traction as a community-based participatory research method, particularly due to its focus on engaging marginalised groups and communities. For instance, Bisung et al. (2015) employed photovoice in a study involving eight Kenyan women to explore their experiences with water consumption, sanitation, and hygiene behaviours. This approach not only facilitated the identification of community-driven solutions to water-related health issues but also served as a means of communicating the findings to the local government and health officials to raise awareness and support policy change.

Photovoice is especially well-suited to research in cultural communities where language barriers may hinder traditional data collection methods. For this reason, photovoice has been widely adopted in studies involving Indigenous populations in countries such as the United States, Canada, Australia, and New Zealand. Anderson et al. (2023) outline several advantages of using photovoice in these contexts, including its potential to enhance participant autonomy and its ability to facilitate community engagement through culturally responsive research practices. These benefits are particularly evident in health research. For example, Jones et al. (2013) used photovoice to examine Māori parents' and children's experience of managing asthma, capturing a range of cultural particularities associated with this health concern. The findings from this study informed an advocacy initiative aimed at raising awareness of asthma disparities and promoting health equity within the Māori population.

However, while photography can help address cultural issues in health research, the use of photographic techniques like photovoice must be approached with cultural sensitivity. In some Indigenous communities, for instance, there are beliefs that photography can "steal the soul", leading to reluctance among some individuals to be photographed or take pictures themselves. Strother (2013) offers a more detailed interpretation of this belief and associated cultural norms that must be carefully considered as part of the reflexive process in photography-based research.

While the idea of empowering research participants through photography is compelling, and photovoice appears to be an ideal method for this purpose – particularly in light of its documented benefits – it is important to approach such methodologies with critical reflection.

Photovoice offers researchers a creative and innovative means of conducting health research, potentially distinguishing their work within the academic field. However, there is a risk of becoming overly invested in the terminology and perceived promise of the method without fully considering its alignment with the specific aims and ethical dimensions of a given study.

In reviewing the literature, I encountered several studies in which photovoice was used interchangeably with photo-elicitation, despite the research objectives being primarily focused on understanding health phenomena rather than promoting social change. This distinction raised important questions at the outset of my doctoral research. Initially, I was captivated by the photovoice methodology, which I familiarised myself with through extensive literature reviews, training, and engagement with experts in the field. Given the sensitive and critical nature of my research – exploring experiences and meanings of recovery from mental distress in a cultural context – I was confident that photovoice would serve as an ideal core methodology. My rationale was grounded in several factors: the need for alternative, non-verbal modes of communication when researching mental distress; the marginalised status of the community where I intended to conduct the study; and my own implicit desire to challenge and transform mental health practices in my home country, Romania, many of which remain oppressive and insufficiently person-centred.

However, this vision was challenged during my initial meeting with participants, who expressed concerns that the use of photovoice – and their potential role as agents of change – might expose them to increased vulnerability and emotional distress. Although this response was initially disappointing, I respected their perspective and began to reflect critically on the gap between my methodological aspirations and the ethical realities of implementation. Through dialogue and negotiation with participants, we eventually agreed to adapt the project to a smaller-scale photo-elicitation study conducted within the safer context of their day centre, rather than extending into the broader community.

This experience was a key lesson in my development as a visual researcher. It underscored the importance of making methodological decisions by genuinely involving the research participants, in keeping with the participatory ethos of the research. Such decisions require ongoing negotiation of boundaries from the onset of the research, along with clarification of roles, discussion of expectations and outcomes, and critical attention to potential power dynamics. These considerations are essential to ensuring that visual methodologies such as photovoice are not only theoretically sound but also ethically and culturally appropriate in practice.

While these reflections may appear to champion noble goals – namely, to prioritise participant-centred approaches over researcher-imposed photographic methods – they are often challenging to implement into practice. One contributing factor is the lack of consistent, standardised guidance on how to conduct photovoice research, alongside conceptual ambiguity that surrounds the terminology used to describe various photographic techniques. Such ambiguity is perhaps unsurprising, given that photography is inherently a creative and interpretive mode of inquiry. Imposing rigid methodological frameworks may risk undermining the very flexibility and innovation that make visual methods so valuable in participatory research.

Nevertheless, the methodological steps outlined by Wang (1999) and Wang and Burris (1997), as outlined in Table 2.2, offer a blueprint that can be adapted by researchers to align with the specific aims and contextual demands of their studies.

The discussion of photographs during photovoice sessions often yields rich, insightful dialogue that can significantly deepen understanding of the research topic. These conversations can be intellectually stimulating and emotionally resonant, offering participants a powerful means

TABLE 2.2 Guidance on conducting a photovoice study (adapted from Wang, 1999; Wang & Burris, 1997)

- Identify and engage a target audience of community leaders, stakeholders, and policymakers who may act on the findings.
- Recruit a group of photovoice participants, typically between 7–10 people, from the community of interest.
- Introduce the photovoice methodology to participants and facilitate an initial group discussion to build rapport and shared understanding.
- Obtain informed consent, ensuring participants are fully aware of the research aims, processes, and potential risks.
- Pose an initial theme or guiding question to direct participants' photographic exploration.
- Distribute cameras and provide clear instructions on their use, including ethical considerations around photographing others.
- Allow time for photo-documentation, typically one week following the initial workshop, to enable participants to capture images relevant to the research.
- Facilitate focus group discussions using the SHOWED method (see Table 2.3) to collaboratively interpret the photographs and identify emergent themes.
- Plan dissemination strategies with participants to share their photographs and narratives with relevant audiences, such as through exhibitions, digital platforms, or community forums.

of expression. However, for novice researchers, and at times even for participants, the process can be disorienting, particularly when uncertainty arises about how to interpret or speak about the images.

To address this challenge, Wang (1999) introduced the SHOWED mnemonic as a guiding framework for facilitating critical dialogue around participant-generated photographs (see Table 2.3). This structured set of questions is designed to prompt reflection, elicit meaning, and support the co-construction of knowledge within the group. Despite its utility, the application of the SHOWED method varies across photovoice studies. Some researchers adapt the questions to better suit their specific context, while others may choose not to use the framework at all, depending on the needs and preferences of their participants.

The PHOTO mnemonic, introduced by Ryan et al. (2020), is an adaptation of the original SHOWED method developed by Wang (1999). It was designed to provide a more accessible and flexible structure for facilitating critical dialogue around participant-generated photographs, particularly in health and therapeutic contexts. Table 2.4 provides a breakdown of this technique.

In photovoice research, visual data generated through participant photography is frequently complemented by textual elements such as captions, descriptive narratives, reflective statements, or other forms of written expression. These written components serve to contextualise the images, enhance interpretive depth, and reinforce the messages participants wish to convey. In many cases, participants are naturally inclined to engage in creative forms of writing – such as essays, poems, or short stories – which are often encouraged within photovoice projects as a means of deepening personal and collective meaning-making.

However, the integration of written tasks must be approached with sensitivity to participants' varying levels of literacy. In some populations, limited literacy skills may pose a barrier to written expression, potentially affecting both the quality of data and the inclusivity of the research process. It is therefore essential that researchers conduct a careful assessment of participants'

TABLE 2.3 The SHOWED method (Wang, 1999) (adapted to health experiences)

S	What do you *S*ee here?	Describe the visible elements in the image that relate to your health journey. What stands out visually?
H	What is *H*appening here?	Explain the situation or emotion captured in the image. What aspect of your health experience does it represent?
O	How does this relate to *O*ur lives?	Connect the image to broader health experiences – yours, your community's, or others with similar conditions.
W	*W*hy does this problem, concern, or situation exist?	Reflect on underlying causes – medical, social, systemic, or personal – that contribute to the health issue depicted.
E	How could this image *E*ducate others (e.g., community leaders, policymakers)	Consider how the image can raise awareness, foster empathy, or inform better healthcare practices.
D	What can we *D*o about the problem or situation?	Suggest actions, changes, or supports that could improve the health experience shown in the image.

TABLE 2.4 The PHOTO mnemonic (Ryan et al., 2020)

P	Describe your *P*icture	Begin by identifying and describing what is visually present in the photograph. What does the image show?
H	What is *H*appening in your picture?	Reflect on the context, story, or emotion behind the image. What moment or experience does it capture?
O	Why did you take a picture *O*f this?	Share your motivation or intention in capturing the image. Why was this moment or subject meaningful to you?
T	What does this picture *T*ell us about your life?	Explore the personal or social significance of the image. What does it reveal about your health journey or lived experience?
O	How can this picture provide *O*pportunities to improve life or help others?	Consider how the image might inspire action, raise awareness, or support others facing similar health challenges.

literacy prior to incorporating writing tasks into the photovoice methodology, ensuring that all forms of participation remain accessible and empowering.

One of the most dynamic and impactful stages of a photovoice project is the dissemination of findings. Central to the ethos of photovoice is the imperative that the voices captured through participants' photographs are not only documented but also meaningfully shared with relevant audiences. Without such dissemination, the potential for advocacy and social change may remain unfulfilled, and the broader aims of the research being addressed only superficially or in a tokenistic manner (Oliffe et al., 2024).

Dissemination strategies such as organising community or online exhibitions, developing dedicated websites, or employing other creative platforms (discussed in more detail in Chapter 6) offer valuable opportunities to demonstrate the impact of the research at both community and policy levels. This is particularly crucial in the context of funded projects, where demonstrable impact is often a key requirement. While such initiatives may introduce additional ethical considerations, as discussed in Chapter 7, they can also be deeply empowering for participants. By making their concerns visible to local stakeholders and decision-makers, participants take an active role in initiating dialogue and informing change.

This emphasis on visibility and advocacy is one of the reasons photovoice has been widely adopted as a strategy in health promotion worldwide (Wang et al., 1998; Ardiles et al., 2019). A notable example is the study by Brazg et al. (2011), which embedded photovoice within the "Our Community in Focus" project to engage U.S. high school students in assessing and addressing substance misuse. Such initiatives exemplify the transformative and empowering nature of photovoice when dissemination is thoughtfully planned and ethically grounded.

To conclude this section, it is important to underscore the participatory value of photovoice as a methodological approach for addressing health inequalities – defined by the World Health Organization (2018) as differences in health status among population groups, often resulting from the inequitable distribution of health resources and limited access to care. Research plays a critical role in tackling these disparities by illuminating the structural and social determinants that contribute to unequal health outcomes among marginalised populations. For example, Jurkowski and Paul-Ward (2007) employed photovoice as an advocacy tool to highlight health promotion disparities experienced by Latino individuals with intellectual disabilities. This study exemplifies the real-world applicability of photographic methods and their potential to influence both health outcomes and policy discourse in meaningful ways.

More recently, the participatory dimension of photovoice has been further enhanced through the integration of co-production methodologies. Co-production is defined by the National Institute for Health Research (NIHR, 2021) as "an approach in which researchers, practitioners and members of the public work together, sharing power and responsibility from the start to the end of the project, including the generation of knowledge" (p. 4). This approach aligns closely with the foundational principles of photovoice featured in research projects conducted *with* and *for* the benefit of research participants and the communities they represent.

Both co-production and photovoice emphasise collaboration, shared ownership, and the prioritisation of participant voices in the research process. It is therefore not a coincidence they are used in conjunction, as illustrated in Barry et al.'s (2021) study engaging service users and family members in the co-production and co-facilitation of a mental health education intervention. Their work highlights the flexibility and creative potential of photovoice when used with marginalised groups. It also demonstrates how co-production can ensure that participants retain decision-making power throughout the research process from inception to dissemination. This represents yet another empowering dimension of photovoice, reinforcing its value as a participatory method in health research aimed at social transformation.

2.3 Visual ethnography

Healthcare research encompasses a diverse array of methodological approaches, among which photography can serve as a versatile and adaptive tool, contingent upon the specific aims of the inquiry. Ethnography, a qualitative research methodology focused on the in-depth study of people within their naturalistic and socio-cultural or organisational context, is one such approach where visual methods may be integrated. Typically conducted over extended periods – ranging from several months to years – ethnographic research employs techniques such as participant observation, document analysis, interviews, and focus groups. This immersive methodology enables researchers to metaphorically "step into the shoes" of participants, opening avenues for a deeper empathetic understanding of their lived experiences – an imperative often underscored in health-related research (Savage, 2000).

Several studies exemplify the application of ethnography in healthcare contexts. For instance, Mncwabe et al. (2021) explored the lived experiences of cancer patients within support settings in a South African municipality; Al-Shamaly (2021) employed ethnographic methods to investigate inclusive caring practices among Australian intensive care nurses; and Stajduhar et al. (2020) utilised ethnography to examine the caregiving experiences of families supporting structurally vulnerable populations at the end of life.

Notably, these studies did not incorporate photographic methods – potentially due to the sensitive nature of the research topics or a lack of familiarity with visual methodologies. Nonetheless, it is critical to interrogate the potential of photography to enhance ethnographic inquiry. While in some cases visual methods may complicate the process without contributing meaningfully to the research outcomes, in others, they may offer unique insights.

Visual ethnography has been employed to enrich healthcare research as a methodological extension that includes photography, video, drawing, collage, and hypermedia (a digital format that extends the concept of hypertext by incorporating not just text but also other media types such as images, audio, video, animations, and interactive elements interconnected through hyperlinks). For example, Riley and Manias (2003) utilised photography to examine governance practices in operating room nursing; O'Regan et al. (2019) promoted visual ethnography in radiography research to facilitate a more holistic understanding of clinical practice; and Fahal et al. (2022) proposed an innovative visual ethnographic approach to raise awareness and promote advocacy for mycetoma in Sudan.

Compared to traditional ethnography, visual ethnography presents both distinct advantages and methodological challenges. Davey (2010) offers a comprehensive SWOT (Strengths, Weaknesses, Opportunities, and Threats) analysis of visual ethnography, originally situated within anthropological research, which may nonetheless inform methodological decision-making in health studies. According to Davey (2010), visual methodologies offer rich epistemological and communicative potential, supported by a growing interdisciplinary scholarship and evolving technologies like digital photography and immersive media. These approaches provide a fertile ground for collaboration, reflexivity, and translational impact, bridging academic research with real-world applications. However, the field faces challenges due to conceptual vagueness, methodological inconsistency, and limited cross-disciplinary dialogue. Practical constraints, especially in time-intensive methods like visual ethnography, and the dominance of Western epistemologies further hinder inclusivity and broader applicability.

Lorenz and Kolb (2020), recommended for further reading at the end of the chapter, provide a comprehensive and methodologically grounded account of visual ethnographic approaches within health and healthcare research. Their work explores the integration of visual methods such as photo-elicitation, photovoice, video ethnography, and graphic facilitation, demonstrating how these can be effectively combined to enrich qualitative inquiry. While Lorenz and Kolb's (2020) discussion resonates with key themes articulated by Davey (2010), such as interdisciplinarity, participatory engagement, and reflexivity, they extend the discourse by providing a detailed, step-by-step framework for designing and conducting visual ethnographic studies in healthcare, as illustrated in Table 2.5.

Visual ethnography represents a complex methodological avenue within healthcare research. Its capacity to deepen understanding through visual engagement – whether via photography, video, or other media – offers unique opportunities for capturing the complex real-world of individuals and communities. However, its application demands careful ethical consideration,

TABLE 2.5 Step-by-step approach to conducting visual ethnography in healthcare adapted from Lorenz and Kolb (2020)

Planning	What is the health topic you intend to explore in your study? Who are your gatekeepers, that is, insiders from the group of individuals, communities, or organisation to be studied, who can facilitate access to the population under investigation? What strategies will you employ to recruit participants for the study? How will you ensure the privacy and confidentiality of the participants, and safeguard them and their communities from potential harm? What will be the frequency and nature of your interactions with participants throughout the research process? How do you plan to incorporate photography in your study design?
Orientation	What are participants' initial perceptions or understandings of the study topic? How will you inform participants about ethical considerations, particularly those related to the use of photography, in order to ensure their safety and the protection of others' confidentiality?
Documentation	What strategies will you employ to support and guide participants in the photo-documentation process, enabling them to visually represent their perspectives and lived experiences?
Contextualisation	In what ways will participants' photographs and narratives be contextualised within the broader framework of their personal histories, social environments, and cultural identities?
Reflexivity	What reflective practices will you engage in to critically examine how your own life experiences, values, and assumptions may shape or bias the processes of data collection and interpretation? What emotional responses do participants' stories and visual materials evoke in you, and how might these affect your role as a researcher?
Interpretation	How will participants be involved in the interpretation of their visual and verbal contributions to ensure the credibility, authenticity, and co-construction of findings?
Outreach	What dissemination strategies are you considering to communicate the research findings to broader audiences, including academic, professional, and community stakeholders?
Translation	How do you envision the translation of your research findings into actionable insights for health policy and practice?

methodological rigour, and reflexive practice. As demonstrated by the literature underpinning this chapter and frameworks such as those proposed by Davey (2010) and Lorenz and Kolb (2020), visual ethnography is not simply an aesthetic tool, but a substantive mode of inquiry that can connect academic and real-world contexts. When thoughtfully designed and critically implemented, it holds the potential to generate rich, participatory, and impactful insights into individuals' experiences of health and illness that can inform both scholarship and healthcare practice.

2.4 Photo-storytelling

Narratives have long held a central place in human experience, not only as a source of entertainment but also as a powerful means of conveying meaning. In health research, storytelling assumes a more purposeful role, often referred to as *serious storytelling*, a concept that parallels the notion of *serious gaming*, where digital games are employed for objectives beyond entertainment, such as education or training. The term *serious storytelling*, as articulated by Lugmayr et al. (2017), denotes a narrative form that emerges from a deliberate and reflective process. It is distinguished by its substantive quality, and addresses issues of significant relevance. When accompanied by visual elements, such narratives can further enhance engagement and understanding.

As a methodological tool, serious storytelling has demonstrated considerable potential in healthcare research, particularly in eliciting rich insights grounded in personal experience (Gray, 2009). Although the term itself remains contested – some critics argue that the notion of *storytelling* may imply fictionalisation – it continues to be widely embraced within narrative inquiry frameworks in health research (Haydon & van der Riet, 2017). The appeal of narrative methods in health-related research lies in their inherent capacity to capture the lived realities of health and illness. As Broyard (1992) observed in his reflections on living with cancer, "storytelling seems to be a natural reaction to illness" (p. 21). Narratives serve as a means through which individuals make sense of their experiences and communicate them to others. Building on this premise, researchers have developed storytelling platforms that enable patients and caregivers to share their illness narratives with healthcare professionals. Such initiatives prompt critical reflection and catalyse systemic change (Getchell et al., 2023). Not only do they amplify patient voices, but they also reposition patients as educators, contributing to more responsive, empathetic, and person-centred models of care.

The communicative impact of narrative research is often amplified through the integration of photographs, which can serve both as a starting point for storytelling and as tools for enhancing the accessibility and resonance of verbal narratives (Balabanović et al., 2000). As with other visual methodologies, the terminology surrounding photography-based narrative approaches is diverse and, at times, inconsistent, ranging from *photo-stories* and *photo novellas* to *narrative photography*.

Some authors (Gomez, 2020) argue that the strength of photo-storytelling lies in combining the power of participatory photography (photovoice) with using images to elicit meanings and lived experiences (photo-elicitation). While the classification of photo-storytelling within either photovoice or photo-elicitation frameworks may depend on the specific aims and design of a given study, the core principle remains the same: the use of visual media to construct and communicate meaningful narratives. As Ryan (2016) suggests, this approach elevates the narrative potential of images to convey lived experiences in a compelling and accessible manner.

An increasing volume of studies illustrates the application and potential of photo-storytelling in healthcare contexts. Sitvast et al. (2010) examined the therapeutic use of photo-stories to explore themes of suffering and acceptance, presenting three in-depth case studies that combined photographic imagery with personal narratives. Klein (2021) employed photo-narratives as a means of visualising mental health experiences among individuals with autism, framing the method as a way of "visualising the invisible". Similarly, Koops van 't Jagt (2019) utilised photo-stories in a randomised controlled trial aimed at improving communication between physicians and older adults in Germany. Although participants in the latter study expressed a preference for the photo-story format over a non-narrative booklet, the researchers found no statistically significant difference in outcomes, highlighting the need for further research into the efficacy and impact of photo-storytelling approaches in healthcare communication.

Although the conceptual foundations and methodological frameworks of photo-based narrative research are still in the process of consolidation, the approach is gaining traction within healthcare practice and education. Its relevance is particularly evident in fields such as narrative medicine and narrative nursing, where storytelling is employed as a pedagogical strategy to develop empathy and critical reflection (Milota et al., 2019; Fitzpatrick et al., 2019).

The potential of photo-narratives in cultivating reflective and empathetic healthcare professionals is exemplified in the work of Leyva-Moral et al. (2021), whose study demonstrated that photography played a pivotal role in deepening students' understanding of caring for individuals living with HIV. One participant in this study encapsulated this transformative experience, stating:

> This methodology [i.e., photo-narrative] has helped me look beyond the disease. I liked it a lot because I was able to understand and experience empathy towards people with HIV from different points of view. . . . For me, it was very useful and a very motivating way to put myself in the place of another, especially with the stories.
>
> *(p. 3)*

Such findings underscore the value of photo-narrative methods in bridging cognitive and emotional dimensions of learning, ultimately contributing to more compassionate and person-centred healthcare practice.

Irrespective of the specific aims of a study, the integration of photographs and narratives can be further enhanced through the creation of digital stories – an increasingly accessible practice facilitated by the widespread availability of digital devices and multimedia technologies. While digital storytelling is mostly associated with short-form filmmaking – a medium explored less in this book – it warrants mention as a dynamic and interactive extension of photo-narrative methodologies in health research. Defined as an "arts-based multimedia presentation of a story, often in the form of a narrated video" (Park et al., 2021, p. 2), digital storytelling has demonstrated transformative potential in both healthcare practice (Hardy & Sumner, 2018) and education (Mojtahedzadeh et al., 2021). For readers interested in further exploring digital storytelling, additional resources are provided at the end of this chapter, including West et al.'s (2022) systematic review, which offers a comprehensive overview of digital storytelling as an emerging method in health research.

2.5 Other photographic approaches to healthcare research

The applications of photography in health research extend well beyond the methods discussed so far. Existing literature highlights a range of techniques that share some conceptual and methodological similarities with those previously outlined. Some of these techniques, briefly introduced in this section, will be illustrated in Chapter 6, which focuses on disseminating photography-based research. These methods demonstrate the virtually limitless ways in which photographic practices can be adapted and combined to investigate the complex realities of health, illness, and care.

2.5.1 Photo-diaries

Photo-diaries have emerged as a valuable methodological tool for exploring diverse dimensions of healthcare from the perspectives of both patients and healthcare professionals. This approach typically involves inviting participants to capture a series of photographs over a defined period (often one to two weeks) to document their experiences in relation to a specific research focus. These visual diaries are subsequently discussed in follow-up interviews, although some health researchers have adapted the method for use in focus group settings (Kuo et al., 2020). By offering insight into participants' socio-cultural contexts and everyday environments, photo-diaries are increasingly recognised as a form of contextual method (Rogers et al., 2020).

The literature reveals a range of methodological adaptations, from providing participants with structured prompts to collaboratively designing photo-missions that guide image production. Variations such as photo-books and photo albums have also been employed, particularly in dementia care research, where the method can be tailored to align with individuals' communication particularities and preferences (Tan et al., 2023). Beyond their utility as data collection tools, photo-diaries have demonstrated therapeutic value by supporting autonomy, enhancing self-esteem, and fostering trust (Harrefors et al., 2012). Some examples of photographic diaries can be found in Chapter 6.

2.5.2 Photo-essays

Photo-essays, also referred to as *picture essays* or *photographic essays*, constitute a form of visual storytelling that involves curating and sequencing a series of photographs to construct a coherent narrative around a specific research topic. This method invites audiences on an interpretive journey, using visual imagery to evoke meaning, emotion, and reflection. In healthcare education, photo-essays have proven particularly effective. For example, Quinn et al. (2006a) employed this approach to enhance obstetricians' and other healthcare professionals' understanding of prenatal care while facilitating reflection on patients' lived experiences and perspectives.

The participatory potential of photo-essays is further demonstrated in public health contexts, such as multimedia campaigns aimed at raising awareness of lung cancer (Quinn et al., 2006b). Regardless of the subject matter, photo-essays are often positioned as alternatives to traditional written essays due to their capacity to communicate complex human experiences in ways that text alone cannot achieve. As Crowder and Cartwright (2021) assert, photo-essays possess the potential "to do the work that often words simply cannot" (p. 2).

In a position piece recommended for further reading, Crowder and Cartwright (2021) offer practical guidance for developing ethnographic photo-essays within medical anthropology. Their framework centred on the integration of compelling imagery, concise textual commentary, and a balanced visual layout is readily adaptable to a range of healthcare research contexts, offering a structured yet flexible approach to visual narrative construction.

2.5.3 Photo-collage

Another photography-based method frequently integrated within qualitative inquiry is the photo-collage – a creative technique involving the collation of photographs or photographic fragments to construct a composite image that symbolically represents the research topic. This method often incorporates additional media such as text, painting, drawing, textiles, stencil work, and other artistic elements, resulting in richly layered visual artefacts. The final outputs may take various forms, including multidimensional pages, scrapbooks, or diaries, which can serve as prompts for photo-elicitation interviews.

Digital adaptations of this method have also gained prominence. For instance, Keisari et al. (2021) utilised digital photo-collage as part of an online, arts-based intervention for older adults.

Their findings highlighted the method's capacity to facilitate the construction of life narratives, enabling participants to engage with the research topic through emotionally resonant and embodied experiences, with both therapeutic and recreational benefits. Similarly, photo-collage has been recognised for its pedagogical potential in healthcare education, where it has been used to foster critical reflection and enhance cultural awareness among learners (Ramluggun et al., 2023). Finally, its application in dementia care has shown promise as a tool for therapeutic reminiscence, supporting memory, identity, and emotional well-being (Stallings, 2010). Some examples of photographic collages and techniques can be found in Chapter 6.

2.5.4 Autophotography and self-portraiture

Autophotography is defined by Glaw et al. (2017) as "an ethnographic research method . . . that creates an environment where the researcher and the reader can see the world through the participant's eyes by the use of photography" (p. 2). However, the conceptual boundaries of autophotography remain somewhat ambiguous, particularly in relation to closely aligned methods such as photovoice and photo-elicitation. The term is often used generically to describe visual research approaches in which participants are invited to take photographs on predetermined themes (Vastapuu, 2022), making it difficult to determine whether autophotography constitutes a distinct methodology.

This ambiguity is further complicated by potential confusion with photographic self-portraiture, inferred from linguistic parallels such as the French *autoportrait* or the Spanish *autorretrato*. While some scholars, such as Thomas (2009), describe autophotography as a broad form of participant-generated photography, self-portraiture more specifically refers to photographic representations created by, and depicting, the participants themselves. Importantly, this distinction does not diminish the methodological value of self-portraits in health research. On the contrary, self-portraiture has been shown to enrich narrative inquiry by enhancing participants' sense of agency and supporting identity exploration across intersecting dimensions such as gender, race, culture, and class. This is evident particularly in studies examining illness identity (Halifax et al., 2004) or documenting the lived experiences of patients and healthcare professionals (Tharenos et al., 2019). Moreover, self-portraiture carries a significant therapeutic dimension, as evidenced in the work of Nuñez (2009) and Jo Spence (Dennett, 2011), further underscoring its relevance and appeal for qualitative health researchers seeking to engage with the emotional and symbolic dimensions of lived experience.

Conclusion

Photographic approaches in healthcare research offer far more than aesthetic value; they provide methodological depth, participatory engagement, and epistemic richness. Techniques such as photo-elicitation, photovoice, visual ethnography, and photo-storytelling introduced in this chapter demonstrate the versatility of photography in capturing lived experiences, creating opportunities for dialogue, and amplifying voices often excluded from traditional research. These methods not only generate rich qualitative data but also create spaces for empowerment, advocacy, and therapeutic benefit. At the same time, their application demands critical reflection on ethical, cultural, and methodological considerations, particularly when working with vulnerable populations or addressing sensitive health topics. Rather than viewing photography as a supplementary tool, researchers should recognise its potential to transform inquiry by bridging visual, narrative, and experiential dimensions of health. When thoughtfully implemented, photographic methods can deepen understanding, challenge dominant paradigms, and contribute to more inclusive and responsive healthcare research.

Knowledge check

1. What are the differences between photo-elicitation and photovoice?
2. What are the steps for conducting a photo-elicitation study?
3. What are the questions that guide the SHOWED technique?
4. How can photographs enhance narrative research?
5. What are the strengths and weaknesses of visual ethnography?

References

Al-Shamaly, H. S. (2021). A focused ethnography of the culture of inclusive caring practice in the intensive care unit. *Nursing Open, 8*(6), 2973–2985. https://doi.org/10.1002/nop2.1009

Alsubhi, M., Epton, T., Goldthorpe, J., & Peters, S. (2022). A qualitative investigation of the health behaviours of young children from refugee families using photo elicitation interviews. *Health Psychology and Behavioral Medicine, 10*(1), 1086–1109. https://doi.org/10.1080/21642850.2022.2141245

Anderson, K., Elder-Robinson, E., Howard, K., & Garvey, G. (2023). A systematic methods review of photovoice research with indigenous young people. *International Journal of Qualitative Methods, 22*(1), 1–37. https://doi.org/10.1177/16094069231172076

Ardiles, P., Casteleijn, M., Black, C., & Sørensen, K. (2019). Using photovoice as a participatory approach to promote youth health literacy. In O. Okan, U. Bauer, D. Levin-Zamir, P. Pinheiro, & K. Sørensen (Eds.), *International handbook of health literacy: Research, practice and policy across the life-span*. Policy Press.

Balabanović, M., Chu, L., & Wolff, G. (2000). *Storytelling with digital photographs*. Proceedings of the CHI 2000 Conference on Human Factors in Computing, Hague, The Netherlands, pp. 564–571.

Barry, J., Monahan, C., Monahan, M., Murphy, R., Ferguson, S., Lee, K., Bennett, A., Gibbons, P., & Higgins, A. (2021). "The road we travel": Developing a co-produced narrative for a photovoice project. *Journal of Psychiatric and Mental Health Nursing, 28*(1), 632–643. https://doi.org/10.1111/jpm.12709

Bender, D. E., & Castro, D. (2000). Explaining the birth weight paradox: Latina immigrants' perceptions of resilience and risk. *Journal of Immigrant Health, 2*(3), 155–173. https://doi.org/10.1023/A:1009513020506

Bender, D. E., Harbour, C., Thorp, J., & Morris, P. (2001). Tell me what you mean by "Sí": Perceptions of quality of prenatal care among immigrant Latina women. *Qualitative Health Research, 11*(6), 780–794. https://doi.org/10.1177/104973230101100607

Bisung, E., Elliott, S. J., Abudho, B., Karanja, D. M., & Schuster-Wallace, C. J. (2015). Using photovoice as a community based participatory research tool for changing water, sanitation, and hygiene behaviours in Usoma, Kenya. *BioMed Research International,* 903025, 1–10. https://doi.org/10.1155/2015/903025

Brazg, T., Bekemeier, B., Spigner, C., & Huebner, C. E. (2011). Our community in focus: The use of photovoice for youth-driven substance abuse assessment and health promotion. *Health Promotion Practice, 12*(4), 502–511. https://doi.org/10.1177/1524839909358659

Broyard, A. (1992). *Intoxicated by my illness*. Clarkson Potter.

Bukhave, E. B., & Huniche, L. (2015). Photo-interviewing to explore everyday occupation: Benefits and issues. *Journal of Occupational Science, 23*(1), 96–107. https://doi.org/10.1080/14427591.2015.1070742

Collier, J. (1957). Photography in anthropology: A report on two experiments. *American Anthropologist, 59*(5), 843–859. https://www.jstor.org/stable/665849

Collier, J. (1967). *Visual anthropology: Photography as a research method*. University of New Mexico Press.

Davey, G. (2010). Visual anthropology: Strengths, weaknesses, opportunities, threats. *Visual Anthropology, 23*(4), 344–352. https://doi.org/10.1080/08949468.2010.485015

Dennett, T. (2011). Jo Spence's auto-therapeutic survival strategies. *Health, 15*(3), 223–239. https://doi.org/10.1177/1363459310397973

Epstein, I., Stevens, B., McKeever, P., & Baruchel, S. (2006). Photo Elicitation Interview (PEI): Using photos to elicit children's perspectives. *International Journal of Qualitative Methods, 5*(3), 1–11. https://doi.org/10.1177/160940690600500301

Fahal, A. H., Otieno, L. A., Ahmed, E. S., Kashif, T., Khalid, M., Mahmoud, A. H., Ododo, L., Kyalo, T., & Bakhiet, S. M. (2022). Visual ethnographic documentation: A novel tool for mycetoma awareness and advocacy. *Transactions of The Royal Society of Tropical Medicine and Hygiene, 116*(8), 679–681. https://doi.org/10.1093/trstmh/trac048

Fitzpatrick, J., Rivera, R., Walsh, L., & Byers, O. (2019). Narrative nursing: Inspiring a shared vision among clinical nurses. *Nurse Leader, 17*(1), 131–134. https://doi.org/10.1016/j.mnl.2018.12.002

Freire, P. (1970). *Pedagogy of the oppressed.* Continuum.

Getchell, L. E., Reich, M., Allu, S., Woods, C., Atkinson, T., Beaucage, M., Stalker, L., Sparkes, D., Turner, C., L'Esperance, A., Burns, K., Elliott, M. J., Chiu, H., Rosenblum, N. D., & Sapir-Pichhadze, R. (2023). Storytelling for impact: The creation of a storytelling program for patient partners in research. *Research Involvement and* Engagement, *9*(1), 1–7. https://doi.org/10.1186/s40900-023-00471-0

Glaw, X., Inder, K., Kable, A., & Hazelton, M. (2017). Visual methodologies in qualitative research: Autophotography and photo elicitation applied to mental health research. *International Journal of Qualitative Methods, 16*(1), 1–8. https://doi.org/10.1177/1609406917748215

Gomez, R. (2020). Photostories: A participatory photo elicitation visual research method in Information Science. *Qualitative and Quantitative Methods in Libraries, 9*(1), 47–63. https://qqml-journal.net/index.php/qqml/article/view/588

Gray, J. B. (2009). The power of storytelling: Using narrative in the healthcare context. *Journal of Communication in Healthcare, 2*(3), 258–273. https://doi.org/10.1179/cih.2009.2.3.258

Greco, V., Lambert, H. C., & Park, M. (2016). Being visible: Photovoice as assessment for children in a school-based psychiatric setting. *Scandinavian Journal of Occupational Therapy, 24*(3), 222–232. https://doi.org/10.1080/11038128.2016.1234642

Halifax, N. D., Gray, R., & Hadad, A. R. (2004). Self-portraits of illness: The gift of the gaze. *Canadian Medical Association Journal, 171*(7), 764–765. https://doi.org/10.1503/cmaj.1041199

Hardy, P., & Sumner, T. (2018). *Cultivating compassion. How digital storytelling is transforming healthcare*. Palgrave Macmillan.

Harper, D. (2002). Talking about pictures: A case for photo elicitation. *Visual Studies, 17*(1), 13–26. https://doi.org/10.1080/14725860220137345

Harrefors, C., Sävenstedt, S., Lundquist, A., Lundquist, B., & Axelsson, K. (2012). Professional caregivers' perceptions on how persons with mild dementia might experience the usage of a digital photo diary. *Open Nursing, 6*(1), 20–29. https://doi.org/10.2174/1874434601206010020

Haydon, G., & van der Riet, P. (2017). Narrative inquiry: A relational research methodology suitable to explore narratives of health and illness. *Nordic Journal of Nursing Research. 37*(2), 85–89. https://doi.org/10.1177/2057158516675217

Hurworth, R., Clark, E., Martin, J., & Thomsen, S. (2005). The use of photo-interviewing: Three examples from health evaluation and research. *Evaluation Journal of Australasia, 4*(1–2), 52–62. https://doi.org/10.1177/1035719X05004001-208

Jones, B., Ingham, T. R., Cram, F., Dean, S., & Davies, C. (2013). An indigenous approach to explore health-related experiences among Māori parents: The Pukapuka Hauora asthma study. *BMC Public Health, 13*(1), 1–11. https://doi.org/10.1186/1471-2458-13-228

Jurkowski, J. M., & Paul-Ward, A. (2007). Photovoice with vulnerable populations: Addressing disparities in health promotion among people with intellectual disabilities. *Health Promotion Practice, 8*(4), 358–65. https://doi.org/10.1177/1524839906292181

Keisari, S., Piol, S., Elkarif, T., Mola, G., & Testoni, I. (2021). Crafting life stories in photocollage: An online creative art-based intervention for older adults. *Behavioral Sciences (Basel), 12*(1), 1–23. https://doi.org/10.3390/bs12010001

Klein, U. (2021). *Photography and visual narratives of autism and mental health: A critical perspective on visualising the invisible*. International Visual Sociology Association Conference (online), University of Brighton. https://research.brighton.ac.uk/en/publications/photography-and-the-visual-narratives-of-autism-and-mental-health

Koops van 't Jagt, R., Tan, S. L., Hoeks, J., Spoorenberg, S., Reijneveld, S. A., de Winter, A. F., Lippke, S., & Jansen, C. (2019). Using photo stories to support doctor-patient communication: Evaluating a

communicative health literacy intervention for older adults. *International Journal of Environmental Research and Public Health, 16*(19), 3726. https://doi.org/10.3390/ijerph16193726
Kuo, M.-C., Chen, C.-M. Wu, F.-G., Chen, C.-H., Yin, Z.-X., & Wang, C.-Y. (2020). Use of photo diary and focus group to explore needs for digital disease management program among community older adults with chronic disease. *Health & Social Care in the Community, 30*(1), 926–936. https://doi.org/10.1111/hsc.13241
Kyololo, O. M., Stevens, B. J., & Songok, J. (2023). Photo-elicitation technique: Utility and challenges in clinical research. *International Journal of Qualitative Methods, 22*(1), 1–8. https://doi.org/10.1177/16094069231165714
Larivière, N., Couture, É., Blackburn, C., Carbonneau, M., Lacombe, C., Schinck, S.-A., David, P., & St-Cyr-Tribble, D. (2015). Recovery, as experienced by women with borderline personality disorder. *Psychiatry Quarterly, 86*(1), 555–568. https://doi.org/10.1007/s11126-015-9350-x
Leyva-Moral, J. M., Gómez-Ibáñez, R., San Rafael, S., Guevara-Vásquez, G., & Aguayo-González, M. (2021). Nursing students' satisfaction with narrative photography as a method to develop empathy towards people with HIV: A mixed-design study. *Nurse Education Today, 96*(1), 104646. https://doi.org/10.1016/j.nedt.2020.104646
Lood, Q., Hermansen Østby, R., Hultqvist, S., Edvardsson, D., & Dahlin-Ivanoff, S. (2023). Uncovering hidden abilities for participation in research through photo-elicitation interviews: A view on participatory research with people living in residential care facilities. *Research Involvement and Engagement, 9*(1), 1–11. https://doi.org/10.1186/s40900-023-00422-9
Lugmayr, A., Sutinen, E., Suhonen, J., Islas Sedano, C., Hlavacs, H., & Suero Montero, C. (2017). Serious storytelling – a first definition and review. *Multimedia Tools & Applications, 76*(14), 15707–15733. https://doi.org/10.1007/s11042-016-3865-5
Milasan, L. H. (2022). Photo-elicitation: Unleashing imagery in healthcare research. In K. Hinsliff-Smith, J. McGarry, & P. Ali (Eds.), *Arts based health care research: A multidisciplinary perspective* (pp. 51–67). Springer Nature Switzerland AG. https://doi.org/10.1007/978-3-030-94423-0_5
Milasan, L. H., Bingley, A. F., & Fisher, N. R. (2022). The big picture of recovery: A systematic review on the evidence of photography-based methods in researching recovery from mental distress. *Arts Health, 14*(2), 165–185. https://doi.org/10.1080/17533015.2020.1855453
Milota, M. M., van Thiel, G. J. M. W., & van Delden, J. J. M. (2019). Narrative medicine as a medical education tool: A systematic review. *Medical Teacher, 41*(7), 802–810. https://doi.org/10.1080/0142159X.2019.1584274
Mncwabe, N., Hlongwana, K. W., & Ginindza, T. G. (2021). An ethnographic study exploring the experiences of patients living with cancer illness in support group settings in KwaZulu-Natal, South Africa. *African Journal of Primary Health Care & Family Medicine, 13*(1), e1–e8. https://doi.org/10.4102/phcfm.v13i1.2303
Mojtahedzadeh, R., Mohammadi, A., Hossein Emami, A., & Zarei, A. (2021). How digital storytelling applied in health profession education: A systematized review. *Journal of Advances in Medical Education & Professionalism, 9*(2), 63–78. https://doi.org/10.30476/jamp.2021.87856.1326
National Institute for Health and Care Research (NIHR). (2021). *Guidance on co-producing a research project*. https://www.learningforinvolvement.org.uk/content/resource/nihr-guidance-on-co-producing-a-research-project
Nuñez, C. (2009). The self portrait, a powerful tool for self-therapy. *European Journal of Psychotherapy & Counselling, 11*(1), 51–61. https://doi.org/10.1080/13642530902723157
O'Regan, T., Robinson, L., Newton-Hughes, A., & Strudwick, R. (2019). A review of visual ethnography: Radiography viewed through a different lens. *Radiography (London), 25*(1), S9–S13. https://doi.org/10.1016/j.radi.2019.06.007
Oliffe, J. L., Gao, N., Fernandez, C. C., Sha, M., Yap, C. Y. L., Sharp, P., & McKenzie, S. (2024). Participatory action research and knowledge dissemination in virtual photovoice: Methodological insights. *Qualitative Health Research, 12*(1), 1–15. https://doi.org/10.1177/10497323241290956
Park, E., Forhan, M., & Jones, C. A. (2021). The use of digital storytelling of patients' stories as an approach to translating knowledge: A scoping review. *Research Involvement and Engagement, 7*(1), 1–19. https://doi.org/10.1186/s40900-021-00305-x
Quinn, G. P., Albrecht, T. L., Mahan, C., Bell-Ellison, B. A., Akintobi, T. H., Reynolds, B., & Jeffers, D. (2006a). The photo essay: A visual research method for educating obstetricians and other health care professionals. *The Qualitative Report, 11*(2), 229–250. https://doi.org/10.46743/2160-3715/2006.1672

Quinn, G. P., Ellison, B. B., Bell, M. Y., Caraway, V., Conforte, D., Lewandowski, A., Graci, L., Stafford, V. P., Sapp, A., Shaffer, A., Shimizu, C., Vaughn, E. J., Willliams, C., Jr., Vadaparampil, S. T., & Bepler, G. (2006b). Faces of lung cancer: A multimedia photo essay. *Cancer Epidemiology, Biomarkers & Prevention, 15*(12_Supplement), B26. https://aacrjournals.org/cebp/article/15/12_Supplement/B26/230242/Faces-of-lung-cancer-A-multimedia-photo-essay

Ramluggun, P., Sulaiman, N., & Alshemeili, A. (2023). Picture collage: A pedagogical reflective practice tool for nursing students in mental health practice. *Qeios* (pre-print). https://doi.org/10.32388/U30GJ7.3

Rayment, G., Swainston, K., & Wilson, G. (2019). Using photo-elicitation to explore the lived experience of informal caregivers of individuals living with dementia. *British Journal of Health Psychology, 24*(1), 102–122. https://doi.org/10.1111/bjhp.12342

Riley, R., & Manias, E. (2003). Snapshots of live theatre: The use of photography to research governance in operating room nursing. *Nursing Inquiry, 10*(2), 81–90. https://doi.org/10.1046/j.1440-1800.2003.00166.x

Rivard, S. J., Vitous, C. A., Bamdad, M. C., Lussiez, A., Anderson, M. S., Varlamos, C., Duby, A., & Suwanabol, P. A. (2022). It's not fine: A photo-elicitation study of rectal cancer survivors' emotions and coping strategies. *Surgery, 171*(6), 1480–1485. https://doi.org/10.1016/j.surg.2021.10.067

Rogers, L., De Brún, A., & McAuliffe, E. (2020). Defining and assessing context in healthcare implementation studies: A systematic review. *BMC Health Services Research, 20*(1), 1–24. https://doi.org/10.1186/s12913-020-05212-7

Ryan, L. (2016). Visual communication and literacy. In L. Ryan (Ed.), *The visual imperative: Creating a visual culture of data discovery*. Morgan Kaufmann Publishers.

Ryan, M., Feld, H., & Yarrison, R. (2020). Using photovoice to encourage reflection in health professions students completing a short-term experience in global health. *American Journal of Pharmaceutical Education, 84*(4), 474–483. https://doi.org/10.5688/ajpe7630

Savage, J. (2000). Ethnography and health care. *BMJ, 321*(7273), 1400–1402. https://doi.org/10.1136/bmj.321.7273.1400

Sitvast, J. E. (2015). Recovery in mental health care with the aid of photo-stories: An action research based on the principles of hermeneutic photography. *Health and Nursing, 3*(1), 139–146. https://doi.org/10.13189/nh.2015.030602

Sitvast, J. E., Abma, T. A., & Widdershoven, G. A. (2010). Facades of suffering: Clients' photo stories about mental illness. *Archives of Psychiatric Nursing, 24*(5), 349–361. https://doi.org/10.1016/j.apnu.2010.02.004

Soaita, A. M., & McKee, K. (2020). Researching home's tangible and intangible materialities by photo-elicitation. *Housing, Theory and Society, 38*(3), 279–299. https://doi.org/10.1080/14036096.2020.1738543

Stajduhar, K. I., Giesbrecht, M., Mollison, A., Dosani, N., & McNeil, R. (2020). Caregiving at the margins: An ethnographic exploration of family caregivers experiences providing care for structurally vulnerable populations at the end-of-life. *Palliative Medicine, 34*(7), 946–953. https://doi.org/10.1177/0269216320917875

Stallings, J. W. (2010). Collage as a therapeutic modality for reminiscence in patients with dementia. *Art Therapy, 27*(3), 136–140. https://doi.org/10.1080/07421656.2010.10129667

Strother, Z. S. (2013). "A photograph steals the soul": The history of an idea. In J. Peffer & E. Cameron (Eds.), *Portraiture and photography in Africa* (pp. 177–212). Bloomington: Indiana University Press.

Tan, J. R. O., Boersma, P., Ettema, T. P., Planting, C. H. M., Clark, S., Gobbens, R. J. J., & Dröes, R.-M. (2023). The effects of psychosocial interventions using generic photos on social interaction, mood and quality of life of persons with dementia: A systematic review. *BMC Geriatry, 23*(1), 1–17. https://doi.org/10.1186/s12877-023-04270-w

Tharenos, C., Hayden, A., & Cook, E. (2019). Resident self-portraiture: A reflective tool to explore the journey of becoming a doctor. *Journal of Medical Humanities, 40*(1), 1–23. https://doi.org/10.1007/s10912-018-9545-x

Thomas, M. E. (2009). *Auto-photography*. Ohio State University.

Vastapuu, L. (2022). Auto-photography. In O. P. Richmond & G. Visoka (Eds.), *The Palgrave encyclopaedia of peace and conflict studies*. Palgrave Macmillan.

Wang, C. C. (1999). Photovoice: A participatory action research strategy applied to women's health. *Journal of Women's Health, 8*(2), 185–192. https://doi.org/10.1089/jwh.1999.8.185

Wang, C. C., & Burris, M. A. (1994). Empowerment through photo novella: Portraits of participation. *Health Education Quarterly, 21*(2), 171–186. https://doi.org/10.1177/109019819402100204

Wang, C. C., & Burris, M. A. (1997). Photovoice: Concept, methodology, and use for participatory needs assessment. *Health Education & Behavior, 24*(3), 369–387. https://doi.org/10.1177/109019819702400309

Wang, C. C., Yi, W. K., Tao, Z. W., & Carovano, K. (1998). Photovoice as a participatory health promotion strategy. *Health Promotion International, 13*(1), 75–86. https://doi.org/10.1093/heapro/13.1.75

World Health Organization (WHO). (2018). *Health inequities and their causes*. https://www.who.int/news-room/facts-in-pictures/detail/health-inequities-and-their-causes

Further reading

Crowder, J. W., & Cartwright, E. (2021). Thinking through the photo essay: Observations for medical anthropology. *Medicine Anthropology Theory, 8*(1), 1–13. https://doi.org/10.17157/mat.8.1.5110

Lorenz, L., & Kolb, B. (2020). Visual ethnography in health and healthcare. Concepts, steps, and good practices. In P. Hackett & C. Hayre (Eds.), *Handbook of ethnography in healthcare research* (pp. 167–180). Taylor & Francis Group.

West, C. H., Rieger, K. L., Kenny, A., Chooniedass, R., Mitchell, K. M., Winther Klippenstein, A., Zaborniak, A.-R., Demczuk, L., & Scott, S. D. (2022). Digital storytelling as a method in health research: A systematic review. *International Journal of Qualitative Methods, 21*(1), 1–25. https://doi.org/10.1177/16094069221111118

3

STARTING A PHOTOGRAPHY-BASED HEALTH RESEARCH STUDY

3.1 Formulating the research question

The prospect of designing and conducting a photography-based study may be exciting. However, it can easily become a complex and discouraging endeavour, if the research question is not carefully formulated and the study's aims and objectives are not clearly defined from the outset. Even when a research idea appears innovative and its intended outcomes are evident to the researcher, it may fail to resonate with funding bodies, academic peers, or supervisory committees unless it is articulated through a well-constructed research question.

Developing a well-formulated research question is critical, as it serves as a guiding lens throughout the study. Many methodological decisions depend on the clarity and structure of this question. For instance, its formulation can indicate the type of knowledge being sought and, in turn, inform the most appropriate methods for data collection and analysis. This includes determining whether photography is indeed an essential component of the research methodology or whether alternative approaches may be more suitable.

Researchers are not expected to formulate a perfect research question from the outset. In qualitative research especially, question development is often an iterative process, as findings may emerge in unexpected and flexible ways compared to more structured experimental designs. Despite its importance, this stage is frequently treated superficially by researchers and students alike. This tendency is often driven by the pressure to make rapid progress, frequently under tight deadlines, without fully appreciating that a poorly defined question may necessitate substantial revisions mid-study. Such revisions can compromise the coherence of the research or require restarting the design process entirely. It is therefore unsurprising that some scholars, such as Riva et al. (2012), recommend dedicating up to one-third of the entire research timeline, from idea conception to publication, to refining the research question.

In my experience as a student and early career researcher, I occasionally underestimated the importance of carefully crafting the research question. This oversight often required me to revise or clarify the question during the publication process. This is a common issue that may contribute to the estimated 30% of articles submitted for journal publication requiring substantial

DOI: 10.4324/9781003537540-4

rewording of their research questions (Mayo et al., 2013). Poorly formulated research questions often stem from a lack of clarity regarding the investigators' core objectives, which in turn compromises the overall rigour of the study (Mayo et al., 2013). It is therefore understandable that tools such as the Critical Appraisal Skills Programme (CASP, 2018) include clarity of aim and research question as the first criterion for assessing methodological quality.

For health professionals and researchers, formulating a research question should not differ significantly from articulating a clinical question in healthcare practice. Regardless of one's clinical background, a variety of scholarly frameworks have been developed to support the effective construction of research questions across diverse study designs, many of which can be adapted to photography-based research. The examples presented in this section focus specifically on photographic methodologies, aiming to guide readers in developing best practices for integrating photography into the formulation of research questions, aims, and objectives.

One of the most widely adopted frameworks for developing research questions is PICO, which stands for Population/Problem/Patient, Intervention, Comparator, and Outcome. Several derivatives of this model exist, including PICOT (which incorporates a Timeframe), PIO (which omits the Comparator and Timeframe), and PICo (Population/Patient/Problem, Intervention/Interest, Context). However, not all studies involve an intervention. In such cases, particularly in qualitative research, alternative frameworks such as PEO – Population/Patient/Problem, Exposure/Experience, Outcome – may be more appropriate. Table 3.1 presents some examples that can serve as a foundation for formulating research questions utilising different frameworks across a range of photography-based study designs.

When formulating a research question, it is important to distinguish between the concepts of *Exposure/Experience* and *Intervention.* In the PEO framework, *Exposure* or *Experience* typically refers to naturally occurring phenomena such as environmental conditions, behaviours, or lived experiences that are not manipulated by the researcher. In contrast, the *Intervention* component in frameworks like PIO refers to a deliberate action introduced or controlled within the research process. For example, casually taking photographs with a smartphone or sharing them on social media may be considered an exposure, whereas participating in structured weekly

TABLE 3.1 Examples of research questions for photographic studies utilising PICOT, PICO, PIO, and PEO frameworks

PICOT	In adult patients with post-traumatic stress disorder (P), how does using guided therapeutic photography sessions to express traumatic experiences (I) compared to standard talking therapies (C) affect emotional well-being and self-expression (O) over a period of 12 weeks (T)?
PICO	In adult patients with post-traumatic stress disorder (P), how does using guided therapeutic photography sessions to express traumatic experiences (I) compared to standard talking therapies (C) affect emotional well-being and self-expression (O)?
PIO	In adult patients with post-traumatic stress disorder (P), how does using guided therapeutic photography sessions to express traumatic experiences (I) affect emotional well-being and self-expression (O)?
PEO	In adult patients with post-traumatic stress disorder (P), how does casual photo-sharing and interaction on Instagram (E) impact their emotional well-being and self-expression (O)?

photography workshops with guided assignments and facilitated group discussions would constitute an intervention.

Photography has been employed as an intervention across a range of healthcare studies, serving both therapeutic and educational purposes. For instance, Calha et al. (2019) used photography as a means of capturing data related to quality of life, which can inform the planning of health interventions for older adults. In a review of nursing literature, Riley and Manias (2004) identified additional applications of photography, including its use as a therapeutic approach and as an educational tool. More recently, Brewster and Cox (2019) conducted an online ethnographic study examining digital photography practices such as "one-photo-a-day" activities as a form of self-care, highlighting their potential to enhance emotional well-being.

While photography is occasionally employed as a therapeutic intervention, it is more commonly used by health researchers as a method for data collection. In a scoping review, Alves et al. (2021) found that the majority of photography-based qualitative studies in healthcare originate within the field of nursing, although other disciplines such as medicine and public health are also represented. In many cases, photography is not explicitly designed to influence health outcomes, but rather serves as a tool for eliciting rich, in-depth data to address research questions. Nonetheless, photography may also hold unintended therapeutic benefits for participants, even when not introduced as a formal intervention (Milasan, 2024).

In the context of qualitative and mixed methods research, alternative frameworks such as SPIDER (Sample, Phenomenon of Interest, Design, Evaluation, and Research type) may be more appropriate for formulating research questions. Unlike PICO, which is typically suited to quantitative and intervention-based studies, SPIDER is designed to accommodate the exploratory and interpretive nature of qualitative inquiry (Cooke et al., 2012).

Table 3.2 presents an example of how the SPIDER framework was applied to structure a research question, adapted from my doctoral research (Milasan, 2020). This framework guided key aspects of the study design, including participant selection criteria and the choice of data collection and analysis methods. Notably, the *Sample* component in SPIDER corresponds closely to the *Population* element in PICO; the *Phenomenon of Interest* aligns with the *Intervention* in PIO or the *Exposure/Experience* in PEO; and the *Evaluation* component is conceptually similar to the *Outcome* in PICO.

In addition to SPIDER, several other frameworks have been proposed to support the formulation of research questions in healthcare. One such model is SPICE (Setting, Population/Perspective, Intervention, Comparison, Evaluation) recommended by Booth (2006) for qualitative research. Another is FINER (Feasible, Interesting, Novel, Ethical, Relevant), which offers a broad evaluative lens applicable across various research methodologies (Goldschmidt & Matthews, 2022). The ECLIPSE framework (Expectation, Client group, Location, Impact, Professionals, Service) is also commonly used in health policy and service management research (Wildridge & Bell, 2002). While these frameworks can provide valuable guidance in articulating research questions, their relevance to photography-based research may depend on the specific aims, context, and methodological orientation of the study.

Regardless of the framework employed, feasibility remains a fundamental criterion when formulating a research question. In healthcare research, ensuring that a question is feasible means it can be effectively addressed within the constraints of available resources, time, and contextual limitations. A well-formulated research question should effectively balance ambition and practicality, taking into account key factors, such as accessibility of the target population, the projected timeframe for data collection and analysis, availability of resources (including

TABLE 3.2 Example of research questions formulated using the SPIDER framework (Cooke et al., 2012)

Research question: What are the subjective experiences and perceived meanings of recovery from mental distress expressed by mental health service users participating in fortnightly photographic workshops over a six-month period?		
Sample	What group of people is studied? (e.g., patients with a certain condition, health professionals, etc.)	Mental health service users
Phenomenon of Interest	What is the topic of research? (e.g., experiences of health)	Lived experiences and personal meanings of recovery from mental distress
Design	What techniques are used to collect qualitative data for investigating the phenomenon of interest? (e.g., interviews, focus groups, observation, etc.)	Participatory photographic workshops combined with photo-elicitation interviews
Evaluation	What is the outcome described in the study? (e.g., participants' experience or perception of the phenomenon)	Participants' perceptions and narrative expressions of recovery through photography
Research type	What is the nature of the research? (e.g., quantitative, qualitative, mixed-methods, etc.)	Qualitative, experiential inquiry using visual and narrative methods

photographic equipment, if applicable), and the level of research expertise (e.g., novice versus experienced investigators). Thoroughly assessing feasibility at the outset of a study helps to prevent delays, minimise resource inefficiencies, and avoid ethical complications. It also contributes to the overall methodological soundness and relevance of the research, thereby laying the groundwork for meaningful and credible findings.

3.2 Research aim and objectives

Once the research question has been formulated, the researcher may choose to articulate the study's aim, which defines the overarching purpose and intended outcomes of the research. However, some researchers may choose to begin with a clearly defined aim, from which the research question is subsequently derived. Regardless of the sequence, a well-defined aim significantly facilitates the research process. Achieving such clarity often requires iterative refinement, similar to the development of the research question. Employing a structured framework such as the SMART criteria (Specific, Measurable, Achievable, Relevant, and Time-bound) can be particularly effective when adapted to the project's scope and objectives.

Building on the research question in Table 3.2, the aim can be formulated as follows:

> To explore the subjective experiences and perceived meanings of recovery from mental distress expressed by mental health service users participating in fortnightly photographic workshops over a six-month period.

This aim is specific and clearly focused on the concept of mental health recovery. However, it could be further narrowed down by delineating particular forms of mental distress, such as depression, anxiety, trauma, or psychosis, to enhance its precision. The aim appears achievable within the proposed timeframe, suggesting it is realistic. Nevertheless, the measurability of such qualitative aims remains a point of contention. In this context, concepts such as data saturation used to determine the adequacy and rigour of data collection may serve as more appropriate indicators of whether the aim has been met (Given, 2008). These methodological considerations are explored in greater detail in the following chapters that break down the steps involved in conducting photography-based research.

Research objectives should logically derive from the overarching aim of the study. While the aim typically addresses *what* the research seeks to achieve, the objectives clarify *how* this will be accomplished. In the context of the above photography-based study exploring experiences of recovery from mental distress, the following objectives can be formulated:

(1) To identify, through participant-generated photography, the subjective experiences and perceived meanings associated with recovery from mental distress;
(2) To examine participants' photographs for potential socio-economic and cultural dimensions that may shape or influence recovery;
(3) To explore participants' perspectives on the potential of photography as a medium to support and promote recovery.

Once the research question, aim, and objectives have been clearly established, the transition to the methodological framework is facilitated by identifying the type of knowledge required to address the research question. This process involves constructing a coherent methodological plan in which the role of photography as a research method is explicitly articulated and theoretically grounded.

3.3 Sampling strategies and participant recruitment

With the methodological plan in place and the role of photography clearly defined, attention now turns to the practical considerations of sampling and participant recruitment – key components in ensuring the study's empirical robustness and relevance.

Subject to a favourable ethical review, the researcher will proceed to initiate the recruitment of participants based on a predefined selection criteria designed to ensure the inclusion of information-rich cases. This stage is critical to the success of data collection and the overall progression of the study. Therefore, it should not be approached as a formality – a tendency sometimes observed in clinical research, where participant selection lacks transparency and depth (Newington & Metcalfe, 2014). In contrast, the justification for selecting a specific sampling strategy must be clearly aligned with the study's ontological foundations – namely, the researcher's assumptions about the nature of reality – and its epistemological stance concerned with how knowledge is acquired and understood. It should also be coherently integrated into the broader methodological framework of the research (Campbell et al., 2020).

In a systematic review on the use of photography as a research method (Milasan et al., 2020), I highlighted the predominance of two primary sampling strategies commonly employed in photovoice and photo-elicitation studies: purposive sampling and convenience sampling. These approaches are further examined in this section alongside snowball sampling that has gained increasing relevance, particularly with the growing use of social media platforms. Although less common in photographic research, probability sampling methods – such as random sampling occasionally used in quantitative designs – are also touched upon in this section.

3.3.1 Purposive sampling

Purposive (or purposeful) sampling is a non-probabilistic strategy widely employed in qualitative health research and, on occasion, in quantitative clinical studies (Benoot et al., 2016). It is defined as a method employed to select participants who are best positioned to offer valuable perspectives aligned with the study's objectives (Kelly, 2010). In practice, researchers may seek participants with specific characteristics such as age, gender, socio-economic status, or particular health experiences that are especially relevant to the research topic.

Participants can be grouped according to these characteristics, with a predetermined number allocated to each group to capture diverse subjective health experiences. This approach is known as *stratified purposive sampling*. A related method, *cell sampling*, also involves stratification, but allows for overlapping categories, meaning participants may belong to multiple groups simultaneously. Such approaches are particularly valuable in intersectional research, as they enable the deliberate inclusion of varied social identities and lived experiences. By acknowledging how overlapping factors such as race, gender, socioeconomic status, and disability shape health perceptions, this strategy ensures that the sample reflects the complexity and depth of intersecting perspectives. However, establishing clear and consistent inclusion criteria in intersectional research can be challenging, with ambiguity in selection criteria risking affecting the transparency and replicability of a study.

Building on these strategies, other sampling methods provide additional flexibility and responsiveness to the evolving needs of qualitative inquiry. For instance, *quota sampling* offers greater flexibility by specifying a minimum number of participants required for each category, ensuring that key perspectives are represented. Lastly, *theoretical sampling* enables researchers to adjust the sample or refine selection criteria in response to emerging findings during the research process (Campbell et al., 2020). This adaptive approach is particularly valuable in grounded theory and other iterative qualitative methodologies.

In relation to the research example presented in the previous section, the application of these sampling strategies is illustrated in Table 3.3.

In addition to the general considerations associated with purposive sampling, photography-based research introduces specific requirements related to the visual nature of the method. These

TABLE 3.3 Application of sampling strategies

Purposive sampling	Involves selecting mental health service users with lived experience of mental distress and recovery, who are most likely to provide rich, relevant insights.
Stratified purposive sampling	Participants are grouped by key characteristics (e.g., age, gender, type of mental distress) to ensure diverse perspectives on recovery are represented.
Cell sampling	Allows participants to belong to multiple overlapping categories (e.g., young adults who are also carers or identify as LGBTQ+), capturing complex identities.
Quota sampling	Ensures a minimum number of participants from each key group (e.g., trauma survivors, individuals with psychosis, or with lived experience of bipolar disorder) to include essential perspectives.
Theoretical sampling	Enables refinement of participant selection based on emerging themes during the workshops, allowing the sample to evolve along with the research process.

include participants' interest in photography and their ability to produce images that meaningfully contribute to the research objectives. Such criteria help ensure that participants possess, or are at least willing to develop, a basic level of visual literacy or creative expression relevant to the study. Importantly, this does not imply the exclusion of individuals with visual impairments. On the contrary, photography-based research can be inclusive, as demonstrated by studies involving participants with visual impairments or other disabilities (Lumia et al., 2021; Dassah et al., 2017; Rothenstein & Gooding, 2016). These examples highlight the adaptability of visual methods to diverse participant needs and capabilities.

Participants are not typically expected to have prior expertise in photography – an important point that should be clearly communicated both in the participant information materials and during the study induction stage. Many photography-based studies offer training sessions focused on developing photographic skills, enhancing digital and visual literacy, and explaining the role of photography within the research context.

However, even with training opportunities in place, some participants may find that photography is not their preferred medium for expressing subjective experiences central to the study's aim. In such cases, researchers must respect participants' preferences and, where necessary, explain why they may not be included in the study. An exception to this would be studies that incorporate a mix of methods which allow for comparing photo-elicitation interviews, for example, with other approaches using different creative media or no media at all.

3.3.2 Convenience sampling

Convenience sampling is a non-probability technique often selected for its practical and logistical advantages, particularly in photography-based studies where participant availability, accessibility, and proximity to the research team are important considerations. This method is widely used in clinical research due to its efficiency in terms of time, cost, and resources (Elfil & Negida, 2017).

However, like purposive sampling, convenience sampling is frequently criticised for introducing selection bias and limiting the generalisability of findings when compared to probability sampling strategies such as random sampling. While studies employing convenience sampling may achieve high internal validity, i.e., the study design effectively measures what it intends to within the sample, their external validity, i.e., the extent to which findings can be generalised beyond the study sample to other populations, settings, or contexts, is often constrained (Andrade, 2021).

Additionally, convenience sampling may introduce motivation bias, whereby the sample is disproportionately composed of individuals who are highly motivated to share particular viewpoints or preferences, such as an enthusiasm for photography. This can lead to the underrepresentation of more moderate or less expressive perspectives, potentially distorting the findings and limiting the diversity of insights captured (Stratton, 2021).

Despite its limitations and subjective nature, convenience sampling remains widely used in qualitative research, particularly in studies exploring attitudes, perceptions, and in pilot or exploratory designs (Golzar et al., 2022). Photography-based studies are no exception, as participants may be readily accessible in settings to which the researcher already has access, such as photography groups, artistic communities, or online forums on social media. This approach can support the achievement of research objectives without requiring extensive logistical planning or resources. However, the practical advantages of convenience sampling must be weighed against potential ethical concerns. These concerns become particularly salient when researchers recruit participants from personal networks, such as friends or relatives – a practice that, while not uncommon, can compromise the objectivity and credibility of the research (Brewis, 2014).

3.3.3 *Snowball sampling*

Snowball sampling is a non-probability strategy occasionally used in photography-based research, in which participants assist in recruiting future participants from their own networks. This approach is particularly useful in studies involving marginalised, hard-to-reach, or niche populations such as individuals with rare conditions who may be identified through local support groups and who, in turn, can refer others with similar experiences. This method is exemplified in Labbé et al.'s (2022) photovoice study, which included 30 individuals with mobility limitations recruited through participant referrals. Another effective application of snowball sampling is demonstrated in Molloy et al. (2025), who employed this approach within a multi-method study exploring the health needs of sex workers in Birmingham, UK.

A key advantage of snowball sampling lies in the trust that potential participants may place in peer recommendations, which can be more persuasive than direct outreach from researchers. However, this method also carries the risk of homogeneity, as participants may refer individuals from similar social or professional circles, potentially limiting the diversity of perspectives captured.

The reach of snowball sampling can be significantly extended through the use of social media, which facilitates access to a wide range of hard-to-reach populations. For individuals facing barriers such as stigma, privacy concerns, or mistrust of formal institutions, online recruitment offers a more accessible and less intrusive alternative. As a result, an increasing number of photography-based health studies are being conducted online, where social media platforms can help protect participants' anonymity and safety, particularly when sensitive topics or personal experiences are being explored.

3.3.4 *Probability sampling*

Photographic research is not limited to qualitative designs. Quantitative approaches that rely on statistical methods can also be employed, particularly in studies evaluating the effectiveness of photographic techniques for therapeutic, rehabilitative, or educational purposes. For instance, Tippin and Maranzan (2022) utilised photovoice as an intervention strategy to reduce mental health stigma among 52 post-secondary healthcare students. The authors measured levels of stigma before the intervention, immediately after, and at follow-up, in order to assess the intervention's impact. However, they acknowledged that the use of convenience sampling limited the generalisability of their findings and introduced potential self-selection bias.

To address such limitations, probability sampling strategies like randomisation are often considered in quantitative research. An example is Russinova et al.'s (2014) study, which tested the efficacy of a peer-led, photography-based intervention (anti-stigma photovoice) aimed at reducing self-stigma and promoting proactive coping with public stigma. In this study, 185 participants from multiple sites were randomly assigned to either an experimental group (n=94) or a control group (n=91). While randomisation can reduce selection bias compared to researcher-assigned groups, it also presents logistical and practical challenges related to ensuring adherence to random allocation and managing attrition without compromising the integrity of the design.

Moreover, the quality of randomised controlled trials (RCTs) can vary significantly depending on the level of methodological rigour. In other words, RCTs should not be assumed to be inherently superior to well-designed qualitative studies, despite common criticisms of purposive and convenience sampling. Regardless of the approach taken, researchers should critically acknowledge the limitations of their chosen sampling strategies and consider how these may influence the overall rigour and credibility of their findings.

3.3.5 Recruitment

Although often used interchangeably, *sampling* and *recruitment* refer to distinct processes within research design. *Sampling* involves selecting a subset of individuals from a larger population who are likely to provide relevant information for addressing the research question. *Recruitment* refers to the process of identifying eligible participants from the sampled group based on predefined inclusion and exclusion criteria, and inviting them to participate in the study. This includes providing detailed information about the research to ensure that participants can give fully informed consent (Tsindos, 2023).

A common dilemma at this stage of research design concerns determining the appropriate number of participants, which can vary significantly depending on the nature of the photographic study. Larger samples typically ranging from 25 to over 100 participants are often used in quantitative studies, for example, randomised controlled trials evaluating photography-based interventions in healthcare, with the aim of producing generalisable findings. In contrast, smaller samples of 5–20 participants are more suitable for qualitative approaches, such as photo-elicitation interviews or photovoice groups, where the focus is on depth rather than breadth.

In qualitative research, the proposed sample size may not represent the final number of participants – not necessarily due to attrition, but because of the principle of *data saturation*. This refers to the point in data collection when no new insights are identified in participants' contributions. Data saturation helps determine whether the sample is sufficient: if themes become repetitive early on, the sample may be too large; if new themes are identified as the study progresses, additional participants may be needed. However, identifying this cut-off point is not always straightforward and can vary depending on the research design and resources available to the researcher (Fusch & Ness, 2015).

Photographic studies add further complexity, as visual data may introduce new dimensions to the research topic that require triangulation with textual data. Braun and Clarke (2019) argue that the concept of data saturation is somewhat illusory, suggesting that participants may always have something new to contribute. This perspective highlights the importance of flexibility and reflexivity in determining sample size in qualitative visual research.

An essential component of study design involves the recruitment of participants and the consideration of appropriate incentives – both of which require careful ethical and methodological reflection. Incentivising research participants can be a contentious issue, particularly when incentives are perceived as excessive, potentially compromising ethical standards (Grant & Sugarman, 2004). Many individuals are willing to participate in photography-based studies without any form of compensation, motivated by the opportunity to contribute to knowledge that may benefit others.

However, for some, the use of photography in research can be inhibiting due to concerns about visual exposure, technical skill requirements, or a preference for alternative forms of expression, such as verbal narratives or other visual media like painting or drawing. As a result, some prospective participants may choose not to take part in the study. It is therefore essential for researchers to clearly communicate during the recruitment phase what the project entails, including expectations of time commitment and involvement. Providing detailed information, along with an introductory training session on using photography as a data generation method, can help alleviate participant anxieties.

For example, in my own research, some individuals felt reassured upon learning that no professional equipment or advanced technical skills were required, and chose to participate primarily for the personal learning and social engagement opportunities the study offered. Conversely, one participant opted out of using photography due to anxiety linked to perfectionism, triggered by his perceived inability to capture images as envisioned. In such cases, it is important to emphasise during recruitment that the study is not a photography competition. The focus lies in the subject matter and the critical discussions elicited by the images, rather than on technical aspects such as image resolution, composition, or quality.

Conclusion

It is important to remember that research rarely occurs in isolation. This applies not only to the formulation of the research question but also to decisions regarding the most appropriate sampling and recruitment strategies. Researchers are often supported by a network of experienced colleagues, mentors, peers, supervisors, librarians, and other experts who can offer valuable feedback during the early stages of the research process, before a more complex plan of action is developed.

Before progressing to data collection and analysis, it is essential to clarify the type of knowledge required to address the research question and to identify the most appropriate sources of that knowledge. This stage can be time-consuming, iterative, and may test the researcher's patience. However, if the research question and aims are not clearly defined, they may misguide subsequent decisions such as compromising the recruitment process, which can lead to inefficiencies in time management, unnecessary stress, and potentially a diminished overall coherence and rigour in the research process.

Knowledge check

1. Which of the frameworks for formulating a research question discussed in this chapter for example, PICO, PIO, PEO, SPIDER, etc., is more appropriate for a qualitative study focused on lived experience of physical or mental health difficulties?
2. What are the similarities and differences between purposive and convenience sampling?
3. What are the key advantages of employing snowballing sampling as a strategy in qualitative research?
4. What is the difference between sampling and recruitment?

References

Alves, K. Y. A., Rodrigues, C. C. F. M., Salvador, P. T. C. O, & Fernandes, S. D. M. (2021). Use of photography in qualitative research in the health area: Scoping review. *Ciência & Saúde Coletiva, 26*(2), 521–529. https://doi.org/10.1590/1413-81232021262.41052020

Andrade, C. (2021). The inconvenient truth about convenience and purposive samples. *Indian Journal of Psychological Medicine, 43*(1), 86–88. https://doi.org/10.1177/0253717620977000

Benoot, C., Hannes, K., & Bilsen, J. (2016). The use of purposeful sampling in a qualitative evidence synthesis: A worked example on sexual adjustment to a cancer trajectory. *BMC Medical Research Methodology, 16*(1), 1–12. https://doi.org/10.1186/s12874-016-0114-6

Booth, A. (2006). Clear and present questions: Formulating questions for evidence-based practice. *Library Hi Tech, 24*(3), 355–368. https://doi.org/10.1108/07378830610692127

Braun, V., & Clarke, V. (2019). To saturate or not to saturate? Questioning data saturation as a useful concept for thematic analysis and sample-size rationales. *Qualitative Research in Sport, Exercise and Health, 13*(2), 201–216. https://doi.org/10.1080/2159676X.2019.1704846

Brewis, J. (2014). The ethics of researching friends: On convenience sampling in qualitative management and organization studies. *British Journal of Management, 25*(4), 849–862. https://doi.org/10.1111/1467-8551.12064

Brewster, L., & Cox, A. M. (2019). The daily digital practice as a form of self-care: Using photography for everyday well-being. *Health, 23*(6), 621–638. https://doi.org/10.1177/1363459318769465

Calha, A. G. M., Monteiro, F. J. L., & Hilário, M. I. T. (2019). Photography in the planning of health interventions for the elderly. *Brazilian Journal of Nursing, 72*(4), 940–947. https://doi.org/10.1590/0034-7167-2018-0329

Campbell, S., Greenwood, M., Prior, S., Shearer, T., Walkem, K., Young, S., Bywaters, D., & Walker, K. (2020). Purposive sampling: Complex or simple? Research case examples. *Journal of Research in Nursing, 25*(8), 652–661. https://doi.org/10.1177/1744987120927206

Cooke, A., Smith, D., & Booth, A. (2012). Beyond PICO: The SPIDER tool for qualitative evidence synthesis. *Qualitative Health Research, 22*(10), 1435–1443. https://doi.org/10.1177/1049732312452938

Critical Appraisal Skills Programme (CASP). (2018). *Critical appraisal checklists.* https://casp-uk.net/casp-tools-checklists/

Dassah, E., Aldersey, H. M., & Norman, K. E. (2017). Photovoice and persons with physical disabilities: A scoping review of the literature. *Qualitative Health Research, 27*(9), 1412–1422. https://doi.org/10.1177/1049732316687731

Elfil, M., & Negida, A. (2017). Sampling methods in clinical research: An educational review. *Emergency, 5*(1), e52. https://doi.org/10.22037/emergency.V5I1.15215

Fusch, P., & Ness, L. (2015). Are we there yet? Data saturation in qualitative research. *Qualitative Report, 20*(1), 1408–1416. https://doi.org/10.46743/2160-3715/2015.2281

Given, L. M. (2008). Data saturation. In L. M. Given (Ed.), *The SAGE encyclopaedia of qualitative research methods* (p. 196). SAGE Publications Ltd.

Goldschmidt, G., & Matthews, B. (2022). Formulating design research questions: A framework. *Design Studies, 78*(1), 1–19. https://doi.org/10.1016/j.destud.2021.101062

Golzar, J., Noor, S., & Tajik, O. (2022). Convenience sampling. *International Journal of Education and Language Studies, 1*(2), 72–77. https://doi.org/10.22034/ijels.2022.162981

Grant, R. W., & Sugarman, J. (2004). Ethics in human subjects research: Do incentives matter? *Journal of Medicine and Philosophy, 29*(6), 717–738. https://doi.org/10.1080/03605310490883046

Kelly, S. (2010). Qualitative interviewing techniques and styles. In I. Bourgeault, R. Dingwall, & R. De Vries (Eds.), *The SAGE handbook of qualitative methods in health research* (pp. 307–326). SAGE Publications Ltd.

Labbé, D., Mahmood, A., Seetharaman, K., Miller, W. C., & Mortenson, W. B. (2022). Creating inclusive and healthy communities for all: A photovoice approach with adults with mobility limitations. *Qualitative Research in Health, 2*(1), 1–9. https://doi.org/10.1016/j.ssmqr.2022.100173

Lumia, C. M., Arbour-Nicitopoulos, K. P., Moola, F. J., & McPherson, A. C. (2021). Using photo-elicitation to explore health promotion concepts with children and adolescents with disabilities: A rapid scoping review. *Disability and Rehabilitation, 44*(19), 5708–5718. https://doi.org/10.1080/09638288.2021.1945690

Mayo, N. E., Asano, M., & Barbic, S. P. (2013). When is a research question not a research question? *Journal of Rehabilitation Medicine, 45*(6), 513–518. https://doi.org/10.2340/16501977-1150

Milasan, L. H. (2020). *Recovery snapshots: A photographic exploration of Romanian mental health service users' experience of recovery* [PhD thesis, Lancaster University, Faculty of Health and Medicine]. https://eprints.lancs.ac.uk/id/eprint/149077/1/2020MilasanPhD.pdf

Milasan, L. H. (2024). 'Taking pictures is like treasure hunting': Exploring the therapeutic value of photography as a qualitative research method. *International Journal of Qualitative Methods, 23*(1), 1–20. https://doi.org/10.1177/16094069241236219

Milasan, L. H., Bingley, A. F., & Fisher, N. R. (2020). The big picture of recovery: A systematic review on the evidence of photography-based methods in researching recovery from mental distress. *Arts & Health, 14*(2), 165–185. https://doi.org/10.1080/17533015.2020.1855453

Molloy, E., Tiwana, R., French, B. C., Christie, C., Smailes, H., Taylor, J., & Bradbury-Jones, C. (2025). 'They look you up and down like you are nothing': A qualitative exploration of sex workers' health needs and interactions with UK healthcare services. *International Journal of Nursing Studies Advances, 9*(1), 1–15. https://doi.org/10.1016/j.ijnsa.2025.100392

Newington, L., & Metcalfe, A. (2014). Factors influencing recruitment to research: Qualitative study of the experiences and perceptions of research teams. *BMC Medical Research Methodology, 14*(1), 1–11. https://doi.org/10.1186/1471-2288-14-10

Riley, R. G., & Manias, E. (2004). The uses of photography in clinical nursing practice and research: A literature review. *Journal of Advanced Nursing, 48*(4), 397–405. https://doi.org/10.1111/j.1365-2648.2004.03208.x

Riva, J. J., Malik, K. M., Burnie, S. J., Endicott, A. R., & Busse, J. W. (2012). What is your research question? An introduction to the PICOT format for clinicians. *Journal of the Canadian Chiropractic Association, 56*(3), 167–171. https://pmc.ncbi.nlm.nih.gov/articles/PMC3430448/

Rothenstein, J., & Gooding, M. (2016). *The blind photographer*. Princeton Architectural Press.

Russinova, Z., Rogers, E. S., Gagne, C., Bloch, P., Drake, K. M., & Mueser, K. T. (2014). A randomized controlled trial of a peer-run antistigma photovoice intervention. *Psychiatric Services, 65*(2), 242–246. https://doi.org/10.1176/appi.ps.201200572

Stratton, S. J. (2021). Population research: Convenience sampling strategies. *Prehospital and Disaster Medicine, 36*(4), 373–374. https://doi.org/10.1017/S1049023X21000649

Tippin, G. K., & Maranzan, K. A. (2022). Photovoice as a method to reduce the stigma of mental illness among health care students. *Health Promotion Practice, 23*(2), 331–337. https://doi.org/10.1177/15248399211057152

Wildridge, V., & Bell, L. (2002). How CLIP became ECLIPSE: A mnemonic to assist in searching for health policy/management information. *Health Information & Libraries Journal, 19*(1), 113–115. https://doi.org/10.1046/j.1471-1842.2002.00378.x

Further reading

Rothenstein, J., & Gooding, M. (2016). *The blind photographer*. Princeton Architectural Press

Tsindos, T. (2023). Recruitment and sampling. In D. Ayton, T. Tsindos, & D. Berkovic (Eds.), *Qualitative research – A practical guide for health and social care researchers and practitioners*. Monash University. https://oercollective.caul.edu.au/qualitative-research/chapter/29/

4

PHOTOGRAPHY-BASED DATA COLLECTION TECHNIQUES FOR HEALTHCARE RESEARCH

4.1 Photo-interviews or focus groups?

One of the key challenges faced by researchers employing photography in healthcare studies is selecting the most appropriate data collection method(s). Amongst the available options, photo-interviews and focus groups are particularly prevalent. This section offers a detailed overview of both approaches, aiming to assist readers in making an informed decision about whether an individual or group-based format is better suited to addressing their specific research questions.

4.1.1 Photo-interviews

Research interviews are a primary method of data collection in qualitative studies, employed across a range of methodological approaches such as phenomenology, grounded theory, narrative inquiry, case study, and ethnography. They are essential for the in-depth exploration of health-related experiences, including patient and staff perspectives on healthcare, as well as subjective phenomena such as beliefs, attitudes, and motivations.

Photo-interviews are iterations of traditional interviews that incorporate photographs into the process to elicit deeper, more reflective responses from participants. For example, in a study exploring patients' experiences of chronic illness, participants might be asked to take photographs of places, objects, or moments that represent their daily challenges or sources of support. These images then become the basis for a narrative discussion during the interview, as illustrated in Fritz and Lysack's (2014) study focused on how people integrate self-management strategies into their daily life.

Interview formats range from unstructured approaches, typically employed when the research topic is relatively unexplored and led by the participant, to structured interviews consisting of standardised questions resembling a questionnaire format. Generally, the less structured the interview, the greater the depth of data that can be obtained. Semi-structured interviews often provide an optimal balance between depth and breadth, which likely contributes to their frequent use in healthcare research and other fields (DeJonckheere & Vaughn, 2019).

DOI: 10.4324/9781003537540-5

Regardless of the specific interview format selected, incorporating a visual dimension through photography can further enrich the interview data, offering deeper contextual insights into participants' experiences of health conditions and enhancing the emotional resonance of the interview through image-based elicitation. Moreover, photo-interviews can empower participants by allowing them to shape the direction of the conversation through the selection or creation of images that reflect their lived experiences. This participatory element is conducive to greater reflexivity and more authentic accounts of healthcare experiences.

Interviews have traditionally been conducted in a one-to-one, in-person format at a physical location mutually convenient for both the researcher and the participant. However, alternative formats such as video calls, email exchanges, and telephone interviews have become increasingly common with the advancement of digital technologies. While these methods can enhance accessibility for both researchers and participants, they may also introduce certain limitations. For instance, telephone interviews do not permit visual contact, thereby restricting access to non-verbal cues and limiting the potential for engaging with visual materials such as photographs. Similarly, online interviews may be impractical when the research design involves physical artefacts, such as printed photographs or traditional collage-making, to prompt discussion.

With the growing digitalisation of data and the widespread use of social media as a virtual research environment, there is a decreasing reliance on printed photographs in research contexts. Researchers may instead draw on a variety of photographic sources, including participant-generated images captured during the study or drawn from personal archives stored on smartphones or cloud services, photographs produced by the research team, and images sourced online subject to appropriate copyright considerations.

4.1.2 Focus groups

While photo-interviews focus on eliciting individual perspectives through participant-generated images, group-based approaches such as focus groups or photography workshops draw on the collective experiences constructed through interaction and dialogue among participants. This collaborative dynamic aligns with constructivist paradigms, which posit that knowledge is not passively received but actively built through social processes, shared narratives, and contextual interpretation (Mahoney & Granvold, 2005).

The logistical aspects of organising and moderating focus groups either face-to-face or online, synchronously (in real time) or asynchronously (via email, discussion boards, or online forums) may deter some researchers. However, the depth and richness of data generated through group dynamics and interpersonal exchanges make this method a valuable option for qualitative data collection.

The optimal number of participants in a focus group varies depending on the desired depth and breadth of data. Some authors recommend six to eight participants (Gill & Baillie, 2018), while others suggest a broader range of up to twelve participants (Cortini et al., 2019). For novice researchers or those with limited resources, smaller groups of four to six participants are often more manageable. Over-recruiting by two or three participants is a common strategy to account for potential withdrawals or non-attendance (Gill & Baillie, 2018). The number of focus groups required in a study, as with interviews, should be guided by the principle of data saturation, as discussed in Chapter 3, which indicates when additional data no longer provide new insights.

One frequent ethical consideration in healthcare research utilising focus groups is the presence of power dynamics, which may influence participants' contributions and compromise the integrity of the data (Tausch & Menold, 2016). To mitigate this, Krueger and Casey (2009) recommend forming homogenous groups to promote balanced and unbiased discussion. This consideration is particularly important when the research addresses topics relevant to both individuals and the communities they represent. For example, in Felton et al.'s (2009) study on the experiences of individuals living with mental distress, separate photo-elicited focus groups were conducted with service users and staff to ensure open and equitable dialogue.

Although the terms *focus group* and *group interview* are often used interchangeably, they reflect subtle differences in emphasis. A *focus group* typically refers to a group-based data collection method that centres on interaction among participants, with the aim of exploring collective views, social norms, and shared experiences. In contrast, a *group interview* places greater emphasis on the role of the moderator in guiding the discussion and eliciting responses to specific research questions, resembling a more structured interview conducted in a group setting (Park et al., 2022). While both approaches generate rich qualitative data, the former prioritises group dynamics and co-construction of meaning, whereas the latter leans more heavily on the researcher's agenda and control over the discussion flow.

Photo-elicitation is generally better suited to focus groups rather than group interviews when the research aims to explore shared meanings, social norms, and collective experiences. This is particularly relevant in healthcare contexts where group dynamics can illuminate how individuals make sense of health and illness in relation to others. In contrast, group interviews, which are more structured and moderator-led, may limit the spontaneous dialogue and peer-to-peer engagement that make photo-elicitation particularly powerful. While they can still be effective for eliciting responses to specific visual prompts, they may not fully capitalise on the collaborative interpretive potential of group-based photo-discussion.

4.1.3 Advantages and disadvantages of photo-interviews and focus groups

Regardless of whether researchers employ photo-elicitation interviews or focus groups, each approach presents both benefits and challenges. In many cases, these challenges emerge as the research progresses, further underscoring the importance of making an informed decision regarding the most appropriate data collection method.

One key area for reflection is the depth of insight required. Photo-elicitation interviews are more conducive to personalised and subjective data, as they focus on individual experiences. In contrast, focus groups typically generate broader, collective insights shaped by group-level interactions, which may be influenced by time constraints and group dynamics. Participants may also conform to dominant narratives, potentially leading to less authentic responses, particularly among quieter individuals. For this reason, photo-interviews may foster greater participant empowerment by allowing individuals to select or create images that reflect their personal experiences. In photo-interviews, the one-to-one format can also help build rapport and trust, which is particularly valuable when discussing sensitive health topics, while in focus groups, the presence of peers may either encourage openness or inhibit disclosure, depending on the topic and group composition.

Focus groups allow for the simultaneous expression of multiple perspectives, which can stimulate new insights through interaction with others' thoughts and visual narratives. As a result, preliminary themes may emerge as participants share experiences and photographs, contributing to the development of collective responses to the research question. However, focus groups present challenges in managing overlapping dialogue and attributing contributions, particularly when photographs are discussed collectively. Finally, from a logistical standpoint, while focus groups are generally more time-efficient and cost-effective than one-to-one interviews, they can be more complex to organise, particularly when arranging a time and location that is mutually convenient for both researchers and participants.

4.1.4 Combining photo-elicitation interviews with focus groups

In some studies, photo-elicitation interviews are combined with focus groups or other group-based methods, such as photography workshops, to draw on the complementary strengths and mitigate the limitations of both approaches. However, this should not be viewed as a default solution for researchers uncertain about which method to choose. The rationale for combining these methods should be clearly aligned with the study's aims and design.

In a study I conducted on mental health recovery (Milasan, 2023), I employed a series of photography workshops – similar in scope and structure to focus groups – prior to conducting individual interviews. Early in the project, discussions with prospective participants revealed varying preferences regarding participation in group settings, one-to-one interviews, or both. Practical considerations also played a role, as some participants expressed concerns about attending regular group sessions due to limited availability and preferred a one-off interview. This combined approach enabled me to develop a broader understanding of the research topic during the workshops, which was instrumental in conducting the subsequent interviews. Key themes that initially surfaced during the group discussions were explored in greater depth, clarified, and reflected upon during the individual interviews.

On reflection, the study could have also benefited from reversing the sequence – beginning with photo-elicitation interviews and subsequently conducting focus groups. Starting with individual interviews would have allowed participants to explore their personal experiences in a more private space, potentially surfacing nuanced insights and emotionally resonant themes without the influence of group dynamics. These individual narratives could then have informed the design and facilitation of focus groups, where shared themes could have been collectively explored, compared, and expanded upon.

This approach may have enhanced the depth and authenticity of the data by first grounding the research in participants' unique perspectives before moving into a space of collective meaning-making. Additionally, it could have supported more inclusive participation, particularly for individuals who may have felt hesitant to speak in a group setting without first articulating their thoughts in a one-to-one context. The focus groups, in turn, could have provided an opportunity to validate, challenge, or elaborate on the themes identified in the interviews, leading to a richer and more layered understanding of the research topic.

Ultimately, whether interviews precede or follow group discussions, combining these methods supports methodological triangulation by enabling comparison between individual and collective perspectives. This not only enriches the depth of the data but also strengthens the credibility and interpretive rigour of the research findings.

4.2 How to conduct a photo-elicitation interview?

Photo-elicitation interviews incorporate photographic elements into conventional qualitative interviews to facilitate meaningful dialogue among the participant, the image, and the researcher, with a focus on the topic under investigation. The integration of photographs has been widely documented in the literature for its capacity to generate rich data. Although various terms are used to describe this method, for example, photo-diary, photo-narrative, photovoice, visual storytelling interviews, photo-feedback, image-based interviewing, reflexive photography, and photographic interviewing, these terminological differences reflect the diversity of techniques employed within photo-elicitation research, particularly in healthcare contexts (Kyololo et al., 2023).

However, this methodological diversity has also attracted criticism, particularly concerning the lack of standardisation and rigour. Common concerns include the ambiguity of visual materials, the potential for over- or under-interpretation, and the contextual dependency of image meaning – where interpretation is often shaped by the participant's lived experience, which may not be fully accessible to the researcher (Reid et al., 2018). This section proposes a systematic framework for conducting photo-elicitation interviews, drawing on healthcare literature and examples to outline key stages in the research process.

4.2.1 Preparing the photo-elicitation interview

Before initiating photo-elicitation interviews, researchers should ensure that the use of photographs is clearly aligned with the study's objectives. It is essential to communicate the purpose of both the photographs and the photo-elicitation process to participants. This information should be included in a participant information sheet to support informed consent and to highlight ethical considerations related to image creation and use during the study.

Researchers may choose to provide participants with prompts to guide their photography (Balbale et al., 2014). However, this approach carries the risk of influencing participants' perspectives on the research topic. Similarly, decisions must be made regarding whether participants will be supplied with photographic equipment or permitted to use their own devices (e.g., smartphones). These preparatory choices are critical to ensuring methodological consistency and ethical integrity in photo-elicitation research.

An important consideration when designing a photo-elicitation interview is the source of the photographic material – whether images will be generated by participants or provided by researchers. The most common approach involves inviting participants to take photographs that reflect the research topic in the days leading up to the interview. In studies employing photo-diaries, however, participants may require a longer timeframe to produce relevant visual data. Alternatively, participants may draw on personal image archives, a practice frequently observed in therapeutic photography (Gibson, 2024).

In some cases, particularly when the subject matter is sensitive, complex, or difficult to capture, researchers may choose to supply the photographs themselves. However, Kyololo et al. (2023) caution that researcher-generated images may not resonate with participants, potentially limiting the depth and richness of narrative responses. When participant-generated photography is employed, researchers should provide clear guidance on the number and selection of images to be brought to the interview, ensuring consistency while allowing for participant autonomy.

Based on my research experience, a selection of three to five photographs for a 30–60 minutes photo-elicitation interview typically provides a sufficient foundation for in-depth discussion. This recommendation emerged from interviews I conducted in which participants brought a large number of images, making it challenging to critically engage with each within the allotted time. Extended interview durations may be an option; however, often unsuitable for participants with mental or physical health conditions, or for healthcare professionals operating in time-constrained environments.

To mitigate these challenges, it is advisable for participants to select their photographs prior to the interview. This process can be facilitated through a preparatory meeting with the researcher, which may also serve to complete consent procedures, although such meetings may introduce additional logistical demands. Regardless of the approach, participants should retain autonomy in selecting images, rather than deferring to researchers' judgments about relevance or appropriateness. Researcher-led selection risks introducing bias by privileging interpretations that align with the researchers' perspectives, potentially overlooking socio-culturally embedded meanings that shape participants' understanding of the images.

The process of negotiating image selection can be considered a preliminary phase of data collection, during which participants begin to articulate meanings and perspectives related to the research topic. These early insights may inform the development of the interview guide and enrich subsequent discussions.

Once the photographic content of the interview has been defined, researchers should develop the verbal component, typically in the form of a semi-structured interview guide. If an unstructured approach is chosen, this preparatory phase may be less time-intensive. However, unstructured interviews are generally not recommended for novice researchers due to the advanced skills required to manage and interpret open-ended dialogue effectively (Brinkmann, 2014).

Semi-structured interview guides typically do not include a fixed number of questions, as this depends on the nature and scope of the research. Nevertheless, photo-elicitation studies often incorporate five to ten core questions to guide the discussion of visual material, supplemented by follow-up questions that emerge during the interview in response to participants' reflections (Meo, 2010).

One widely used framework for developing photo-elicitation questions is the SHOWED technique (Wang, 1999) introduced in Chapter 2 (see Table 2.3). While this framework offers a useful starting point for engaging with visual data, it may not fully capture the complexity and richness of photographic material in a health study.

To address this limitation, I advanced an alternative, more comprehensive mnemonic – IMPARTED (Table 4.1). This framework places greater emphasis on the interpretive depth of images and reinforces the distinctiveness of photo-elicitation as a method that prioritises visual inquiry over conventional verbal interviewing.

4.2.2 Conducting the photo-elicitation interview

Conducting photo-elicitation interviews is not significantly different from conducting conventional qualitative interviews, a widely used data collection method in healthcare research supported by an extensive body of literature. For instance, McGrath et al. (2018) offer twelve practical recommendations for novice researchers undertaking qualitative interviews in medical education. This chapter does not seek to redefine established interview practices, but rather to highlight specific considerations that are particularly important when conducting photo-elicitation interviews.

The check-in stage involves welcoming the participant and conducting introductions. At this point, the researcher should reiterate the purpose and scope of the study and provide an overview of the interview process, including the estimated duration – typically between 30 and

TABLE 4.1 Developing interview and focus group questions for photography-based studies in healthcare using the IMPARTED mnemonic

Importance	What makes this photograph significant or relevant to the research topic or health phenomena?
Meaning	What meaning does this image – or specific elements within it – convey with regards to health and/or illness?
Place	Where was this photograph taken, and why is the location important for exploring a health condition?
Aesthetics	How do visual elements such as colour, contrast, lighting, angle, or composition contribute to the image's message?
Reason	What motivated you to take this photograph in relation to the research topic?
Thoughts	What were your thoughts when you captured this image?
Emotions	What emotions did you experience while taking this photograph?
Difference	Is there anything missing from the image, or anything you would have preferred to include?

60 minutes. The length and location of the interview should be adapted, where necessary, to accommodate the needs of individuals with health conditions or other accessibility requirements.

Informed consent must be obtained either in writing or verbally, including parental consent where applicable. Any questions the participant may have should be addressed before proceeding with the interview. Participants should also be reminded of their right to withdraw from the interview at any time and to skip any questions they find uncomfortable.

One critical aspect that must be checked prior to the interview is the functionality of the audio recording equipment. Ensuring that the interview is successfully recorded and subsequently transcribed is essential for accurate data analysis.

Photographs – whether printed or displayed electronically – should be prepared in advance of the interview questions. When exploring photographs, open-ended questions are preferred to encourage reflection, and probing questions may be used to explore deeper meanings, provided they do not lead participants toward specific interpretations.

Periods of silence are a natural part of qualitative interviews and may cause discomfort for both participants and researchers. However, the presence of visual material can help mitigate this by providing a focal point for attention. Reassuring participants that they may take time to reflect on their photographs before responding can also help manage silence and reduce anxiety.

As with any stage of the research process, photo-elicitation interviews may not always unfold as anticipated. For example, researchers may be diverted from the structure of the IMPARTED mnemonic due to unexpected participant disclosures or emotional responses. In such cases, flexibility is essential; adhering rigidly to a scripted format may result in missed opportunities to explore issues that are meaningful to participants. Similarly, participants may occasionally diverge from the research topic. In these instances, photographs can serve as effective tools to reorient the discussion and maintain focus.

At the conclusion of the interview, it is considered best practice to assess the participant's emotional state, particularly if the discussion has involved sensitive topics. In healthcare-related photo-elicitation studies, it is common for photographs to elicit personal disclosures that require sensitive and ethical handling. To support participants, researchers should offer a debriefing opportunity immediately following the interview or, at least, remind participants of the debriefing information sheet provided at the outset of the study.

Before leaving the interview, participants should be reminded again of their right to withdraw their data, and a clear timeframe should be communicated within which this decision can be made. Before concluding the session, researchers should also outline the next steps in the research process. For example, participants may be invited to take part in a feedback and reflection session commonly referred to as member-checking to review preliminary findings and ensure accurate representation of their verbal and visual contributions.

Additionally, it is good practice to ask participants whether they would like to receive copies of research outputs, such as journal articles, conference presentations, or other dissemination materials that include their contributions. This not only promotes transparency but also acknowledges and values their role in the co-production of knowledge. In participatory or co-produced research, participants may also be invited to take an active role in dissemination activities themselves. This could include co-presenting at conferences, contributing to publications, or participating in community engagement events. Such involvement can enhance the relevance and impact of the research and ensure that the findings are communicated in ways that are meaningful and accessible to diverse audiences.

4.3 How to organise photovoice activities?

While photo-elicitation is typically employed in one-to-one interviews as a data collection method to evoke discussions, reflections, and memories, photovoice is more commonly used in group-based methodologies such as photography-focused workshops and focus groups. In photovoice activities, the emphasis is on collective reflection and social action (see Chapter 2 for more information on photo-elicitation and photovoice). However, this distinction does not preclude methodological flexibility. Photo-elicitation can be effectively integrated into group settings (Walstra, 2020), and photovoice principles can be adapted for use in individual interviews (Edwards & Greef, 2017), provided that the chosen approach is underpinned by a clear rationale and that photography is incorporated in a methodologically coherent and purposeful manner.

Photovoice groups can be more challenging to organise from a logistical perspective, yet they offer several advantages over photo-elicitation interviews. These include the empowering nature of photovoice activities. This aspect is key to the collective exploration of health concerns and the identification of solutions – particularly in marginalised or underrepresented communities (Hines et al., 2022).

A further strength of the photovoice approach lies in its participatory ethos; the purpose and objectives of the study are often defined collaboratively from the outset, with participants who are both directly invested in the research topic and positioned as primary beneficiaries of its outcomes. These characteristics introduce several distinctive considerations for organising photovoice groups elaborated upon in the subsequent sections, requiring researchers to remain focused on the participatory and empowering principles that underpin this methodology.

4.3.1 Preparing the photovoice group

The preparatory phase of a photovoice project is often more complex than that of a photo-elicitation interview, primarily due to the logistical demands associated with group-based participatory research. A key step involves developing a schedule that is mutually convenient for both the research team and participants. This includes determining the overall duration of the project, the frequency and timing of meetings, the time allocated for participants to take photographs between sessions, and securing a venue that is safe, accessible, and comfortable for all involved.

The choice of venue should not only accommodate regular group meetings but also anticipate the potential for a community exhibition at the conclusion of the project. In many photovoice studies, the knowledge and visual materials generated through photovoice are frequently shared in community exhibitions or broader dissemination events at the conclusion of the project. These activities aim to amplify the research's impact and raise awareness of the issues explored. However, such dissemination activities also have implications for the time, financial, and logistical resources required to successfully complete a photovoice study, and should therefore be factored into early project planning.

With regard to the equipment required for research purposes, cameras or smartphones may be provided to participants, particularly in cases where individuals come from low-income or socio-economically disadvantaged communities and may not have access to such devices. A preparatory session may also be necessary to introduce participants to the photovoice methodology, including its purpose, process, and ethical considerations for example, obtaining consent when photographing others, and to provide basic training on how to use the equipment (Jongeling et al., 2016).

The literature presents mixed perspectives on whether participants should receive detailed instructions on the types of images to capture and how to interpret the research themes. Regardless of the approach, it is essential to provide participants with a clear photographic focus. This guidance helps ensure that participants remain aligned with the research objectives and do not use photography for unrelated purposes, such as purely recreational, which may reduce the relevance of their visual contributions and limit the depth of subsequent discussions.

4.3.2 Facilitating photovoice group discussions

Photovoice groups should be understood as more than simply a means of bringing individuals together for research purposes. Rooted in participatory and community-based methodologies, photovoice is designed to surface and address concerns that are meaningful to community members – concerns that may not only inform research but also catalyse social awareness and change.

As such, photovoice groups often serve as platforms for representing local perspectives that may diverge from, or even challenge, the priorities of governmental or institutional stakeholders. This dynamic can lead to critical discussions that, in some cases, take on the character of advocacy or protest, amplifying the visibility and impact of the group's collective voice.

Researchers facilitating such groups must be prepared to support these developments, regardless of their own social or political positions. Maintaining a reflexive stance is essential. For this purpose, researchers are encouraged to document their reflections in a research diary, which can later contribute to the qualitative dataset and overall rigour of the study. This practice not only enhances transparency but also supports ethical reflexivity and accountability in participatory research.

Photovoice groups require advanced communication and facilitation skills, which can be supported by involving a co-facilitator. The co-facilitator may be another researcher or a gatekeeper, that is, a key person within the organisation or community where the research takes place. Ledger et al. (2019) provide an excellent example of co-facilitation in a focus group involving patient representatives, who also co-designed the group materials in line with co-production principles. Reflecting on this approach, the authors concluded: "Co-facilitation of the groups enabled transparency, legitimacy and balance of contribution across academic and lay representatives. Rather than following convention and leading a focus group, researchers' roles shifted, and they became co-facilitators" (p. A5).

In addition to supporting the democratisation of the research process, the presence of a co-facilitator can contribute to a safer and more responsive group environment. For instance, if a participant needs to step away due to emotional distress, a co-facilitator can provide support with minimal disruption to the ongoing session.

Given the typical duration of a photovoice session (60–90 minutes) and the average group size of seven to ten participants (Palibroda et al., 2009), it is essential to allocate sufficient time for both individual presentations of photographs and collective critical discussions. Striking a balance between these components can be challenging, particularly when some participants may dominate the conversation or require more time to express their views.

Effective time management and structured facilitation are therefore crucial. Strategies such as a round-table approach can help ensure that all participants have an equal opportunity to explore their photographs and contribute their perspectives on the research topic. These facilitation practices not only support inclusivity but also enhance the quality of group dialogue.

To promote a respectful and productive group environment, these considerations should be formalised in a set of ground rules or a group agreement established at the outset of the project. This agreement can also address additional expectations and responsibilities such as confidentiality, respectful listening, and time-sharing, as illustrated in Table 4.2.

An important stage in the photovoice process involves participants sharing the photographs they have taken. As with photo-elicitation interviews, it is advisable that participants pre-select a limited number of images prior to the group session to ensure efficient use of time during group activities. The selection process itself can offer valuable insights into participants' priorities, concerns, and meanings they attribute to specific images, thereby enriching the researcher's prior understanding of their perspectives.

Dialogue and critical discussion of photographs during photovoice sessions can be effectively facilitated using open-ended questions or prompts like those exemplified in Table 4.3. Additionally, the SHOWED and IMPARTED techniques outlined in the previous section can be adapted to explore the meanings, narratives, and social contexts embedded in participants' images. These approaches help elicit participants' perspectives on how their photographs reflect lived experiences, socio-economic contexts, or health-related circumstances they may wish to challenge or change.

4.3.3 Post-group considerations

Shortly after the final photovoice session, researchers are encouraged to create opportunities for participants to reflect on their experiences of being part of the group. These reflections may include what participants have learned, how they have grown or developed throughout the project, and what the process has meant to them personally and collectively. Such insights are valuable for evaluating the effectiveness of the project and identifying areas for improvement in future participatory research.

TABLE 4.2 Ground rules for a photovoice group

Confidentiality	What is shared in the group stays within the group, unless explicit consent is given to share outside. Respect the privacy of individuals and the stories behind their photographs. Always obtain consent before sharing any photos or narratives beyond the group.
Respect for others	Be open to diverse perspectives and avoid judgment of group members' verbal contributions and their photographs. Allow each person to speak without interruption. Use inclusive, respectful, and non-discriminatory language at all times.
Participation	All members are encouraged to attend regularly and engage actively in discussions. However, participation is voluntary – no one is required to speak or share, if they do not feel comfortable to do so. Time should be shared equitably to ensure everyone has a chance to explore their photographs and contribute their perspectives.
Sensitivity	Be mindful of potentially triggering topics or images. Approach personal or difficult themes with care and empathy.
Constructive feedback	Provide feedback in a supportive and constructive manner. Focus on the message and meaning of the photos rather than technical quality.
Focus on purpose	Keep discussions centred on the topic and aim of the project. Stay committed to using photography as a tool for storytelling, reflection, and social change.
Support	Support and value one another. Encourage learning, skills development, growth, and mutual respect throughout the project.

TABLE 4.3 Open-ended prompts to enhance critical dialogue and ensure that the theme of social change remains central to the photovoice methodology

- Who is the intended audience for key messages generated in photovoice activities?
- Which groups have the capacity to influence decisions?
- Who holds the authority to enact the changes envisaged by participants?
- How would these changes benefit the local community?

If the project includes a photo exhibition or other public presentation of outcomes, researchers should also facilitate a session for participants to curate their photographs and develop accompanying captions or narratives. Regardless of the format of the dissemination event – whether in-person or online – community engagement is essential to ensure participants' photo-stories and key messages reach relevant audiences, for example, health authorities, community leaders, and policymakers.

Community involvement in dissemination can extend the impact of the project by sparking broader dialogue and initiating or strengthening collaboration with external partners, including local or national media organisations. Researchers can also play an important role in connecting participants with networks, organisations, or individuals who may support their future advocacy or creative endeavours. In some cases, participants may be invited to take part directly in dissemination activities, such as speaking at exhibitions or co-presenting findings, provided that ethical considerations such as informed consent and safeguarding are fully addressed. This approach not only amplifies participants' voices but also reinforces the empowering ethos of photovoice.

These dimensions can be incorporated into an impact assessment conducted at both individual and community levels. Community-level impact may be evidenced through increased awareness, shifts in attitudes, policy changes, or other tangible outcomes resulting from the project. It is considered good practice to keep participants informed of ongoing developments and outputs, ensuring they feel valued and included in the project's legacy. Encouraging participants to take on leadership roles in future community initiatives can further sustain the momentum generated by the project.

Celebrating achievements at the conclusion of the project is also important for recognising the contributions of both participants and researchers. This may include offering certificates, awards, or public acknowledgements. Dissemination may continue beyond the project's life through academic publications, conference presentations, or other outputs to which participants have consented to contribute. In such cases, participants typically retain ownership of their visual and verbal contributions unless otherwise agreed.

4.4 Online photography-based healthcare research

The collection of photographic data for research purposes extends beyond traditional methods such as photo-elicitation interviews, photography workshops, and photovoice studies. In recent years, particularly since the COVID-19 pandemic, which necessitated alternatives to in-person research, social media has emerged as a valuable tool in healthcare research and beyond. Initially used primarily for participant recruitment and dissemination of findings, social media platforms have evolved into significant sources of health-related information and visual data. Platforms such as Facebook, Instagram, X (formerly Twitter), YouTube, and TikTok now host a vast array of user-generated content, including images that can offer rich insights into public perceptions, behaviours, and experiences related to health and well-being.

This section focuses on Instagram, a widely used visual social media platform that enables users globally to share photos, videos, and stories in an interactive, image-centric format. As of April 2024, Instagram hosts an estimated 2 billion monthly active users who collectively post approximately 100 million photos and videos each day. This immense volume of user-generated visual content presents significant opportunities for research. Accordingly, Instagram has become a primary data source for a growing number of healthcare studies employing diverse methodologies. These studies have explored topics such as mental health (Adeyanju et al., 2021), substance use (Malik et al., 2022), pregnancy (Jones et al., 2024), nutrition and dietary trends (Tricas-Vidal et al., 2022), physical activity (Liu et al., 2021), sexual health (Nobles et al., 2020), and health inequities (Gonzales, 2022), among others.

Oliveira et al. (2022) provide a comprehensive overview of using Instagram as an infodemiological tool, that is, the application of information epidemiology to monitor and analyse health-related content shared online, with the aim of informing public health and policy. In their study, the authors identified Instagram as a key data source in oral health research. Among the methodologies employed, content analysis of Instagram posts was the most common, followed by frequency-based and other descriptive analytical approaches. The study concluded that Instagram offers researchers access to substantial volumes of visual data, often accompanied by captions and hashtags, at a relatively low cost compared to traditional public health data sources.

The methods used by researchers to access and analyse social media data have evolved in response to increasing platform restrictions. For instance, Instagram permanently disabled access to its Legacy Application Programming Interface (API) in June 2020. While this change enhanced user privacy and autonomy, it also introduced new challenges for researchers seeking to engage with the platform. Mortensen and McCrow-Young (2022) offer a detailed account of sourcing visual data, captions, and comments from Instagram in their study of online mourning rituals following the Manchester Arena attack in 2017. Their approach involved the use of third-party tools alongside a discussion of their limitations and manual strategies to reconstruct and refine datasets. They also provide guidance on data archiving and management in accordance with General Data Protection Regulation (GDPR) requirements. This is particularly relevant given the growing ethical concerns surrounding research involving private or sensitive content, such as substance misuse, mental health, and pregnancy (Golder et al., 2017). Additionally, Mortensen and McCrow-Young (2022) highlight the importance of anonymising identifiable visual data such as through blurring or pixelation of facial features.

This section highlights the complexities underlying research practices often assumed to be straightforward due to the perceived "public" nature of social media profiles. However, public availability does not automatically grant researchers the ethical right to use such data for research purposes. As digital environments, platform policies, and regulatory frameworks continue to evolve, albeit in varying ways across different countries, research methodologies must be regularly reassessed and adapted. It is therefore essential for health researchers to remain informed about these developments to ensure that their study designs and data collection strategies are ethically robust. Further discussion on the ethical responsibilities of conducting online research, along with potential solutions to common dilemmas in photography-based studies, will be presented in Chapter 7.

Conclusion

Photography-based data collection techniques offer healthcare researchers powerful tools for eliciting rich insights into people's lived experiences. Methods such as photo-elicitation interviews and photovoice groups extend beyond traditional verbal approaches by promoting reflection, dialogue, and participatory engagement. Each technique carries distinct advantages: interviews provide depth and privacy for exploring personal narratives, while group-based approaches enable collective meaning-making, participation, and advocacy. Combining these methods can enhance methodological rigour through triangulation, but requires careful planning to avoid tokenistic integration. When implemented with care, these methods can transform healthcare research into a more inclusive, participatory, and visually grounded practice that amplifies voices and enhances understanding of experiences of health and illness.

Knowledge check

1. What are the key advantages and limitations of using photo-elicitation interviews compared to photography workshops or other group-based photographic activities in health research?
2. In what ways might combining photo-elicitation interviews with photographic group activities enhance the methodological design of a photography-based study in healthcare research?
3. What ethical, methodological, and practical challenges arise when conducting online healthcare research that relies on images sourced from visual social media platforms such as Instagram?

References

Adeyanju, G. C., Solfa, R. P., Tran, T. L., Wohlfarth, S., Büttner, J., Osobajo, O. A., & Otitoju, A. (2021). Behavioural symptoms of mental health disorder such as depression among young people using Instagram: A systematic review. *Translational Medicine Communications, 6*(15), 1–13. https://doi.org/10.1186/s41231-021-00092-3

Balbale, S. N., Morris, M. A., & LaVela, S. L. (2014). Using photovoice to explore patient perceptions of patient-centered care in the Veterans Affairs Health Care System. *Patient, 7*(2), 187–195. https://doi.org/10.1007/s40271-014-0044-5

Brinkmann, S. (2014). Unstructured and semi-structured interviewing. In P. Leavy (Ed.), *The Oxford Handbook of Qualitative Research,* pp. 277–299. https://doi.org/10.1093/oxfordhb/9780199811755.013.030

Cortini, M., Galanti, T., & Fantinelli, S. (2019). Focus group discussion: How many participants in a group? *Journal of Phenomenology and Education, 23*(54), 29–43. https://doi.org/10.6092/issn.1825-8670/9603

DeJonckheere, M., & Vaughn, L. M. (2019). Semistructured interviewing in primary care research: A balance of relationship and rigour. *Family Medicine and Community Health, 7*(2), 1–8. https://doi.org/10.1136/fmch-2018-000057

Edwards, L. B., & Greef, L. (2017). Evidence-based feedback about emotional cancer challenges experienced in South Africa: A qualitative analysis of 316 photovoice interviews. *Global Public Health, 13*(2), 1–13. https://doi.org/10.1080/17441692.2017.1357187

Felton, A., Arnold, P., Fairbank, S., & Shaw, T. (2009). Using focus groups and photography to evaluate experiences of social inclusion within rehabilitation adult mental health services. *Mental Health Review Journal, 14*(3), 13–22. https://doi.org/10.1108/13619322200900017

Fritz, H., & Lysack, C. (2014). "I see it now": Using photo elicitation to understand chronic illness self-management. *Canadian Journal of Occupational Therapy, 81*(4), 247–255. https://doi.org/10.1177/0008417414540517

Gibson, N. (2024). Using therapeutic photography in social work – an interpretive phenomenological analysis of the dynamics within a group programme. *The British Journal of Social Work, 54*(1), 305–325. https://doi.org/10.1093/bjsw/bcad196

Gill, P., & Baillie, J. (2018). Interviews and focus groups in qualitative research: An update for the digital age. *British Dental Journal, 225*(1), 668–672. https://doi.org/10.1038/sj.bdj.2018.815

Golder, S., Ahmed, S., Norman, G., & Booth, A. (2017). Attitudes toward the ethics of research using social media: A systematic review. *Journal of Medical Internet Research, 19*(6), 1–19. https://doi.org/10.2196/jmir.7082

Gonzales, G. G. (2022). COVID-19, Black Lives Matter, and healthy food blogs: Individualized approaches to racial health inequalities. *Sociological Spectrum, 42*(3), 176–194. https://doi.org/10.1080/02732173.2022.2081892

Hines, A. L., Brody, R., Zhou, Z., Collins, S. V., Omenyi, C., Miller, E. R., Cooper, L. A., & Crews, D. C. (2022). Contributions of structural racism to the food environment: A photovoice study of black residents with hypertension in Baltimore, MD. *Circulation: Cardiovascular Quality and Outcomes, 15*(11), 869–879. https://doi.org/10.1161/CIRCOUTCOMES.122.009301

Jones, H. M., Orr, J., Whelan, M. E., & Oyebode, O. (2024). An exploration of pregnancy and postpartum content on Instagram: A content analysis of health and exercise focused accounts. *Women and Birth, 37*(4), 1–9. https://doi.org/10.1016/j.wombi.2024.101632

Jongeling, S., Bakker, M., van Zorge, R., & van Kakebeeke, K. (2016). *Photovoice. Facilitator's guide.* Rutgers International.

Krueger, R. A., & Casey, M. A. (2009). *Focus groups: A practical guide for applied research* (4th ed.). Sage Publications Ltd.

Kyololo, O. M., Stevens, B. J., & Songok, J. (2023). Photo-elicitation technique: Utility and challenges in clinical research. *International Journal of Qualitative Methods, 22*(1), 1–8. https://doi.org/10.1177/16094069231165714

Ledger, J., Mehta, R., Jasim, S., Aspinal, F., & Barratt, H. (2019). Democratising the research process: Reflections on the co-production of focus groups. *BMJ Open, 9*(1), A5. https://doi.org/10.1136/bmjopen-2019-QHRN.12

Liu, S., Perdew, M., Lithopoulos, A., & Rhodes, R. E. (2021). The feasibility of using Instagram data to predict exercise identity and physical activity levels: Cross-sectional observational study. *Journal of Medical Internet Research, 23*(4), 1–11. https://doi.org/10.2196/20954

Mahoney, M. J., & Granvold, D. K. (2005). Constructivism and psychotherapy. *World Psychiatry, 4*(2), 74–77. https://pmc.ncbi.nlm.nih.gov/articles/PMC1414735/

Malik, A., Berggren, W., & Al-Busaidi, A. S. (2022). Instagram as a research tool for examining tobacco-related content: A methodological review. *Technology in Society, 70*(1), 1–12. https://doi.org/10.1016/j.techsoc.2022.102008

McGrath, C., Palmgren, P. J., & Liljedahl, M. (2018). Twelve tips for conducting qualitative research interviews. *Medical Teacher, 41*(9), 1002–1006. https://doi.org/10.1080/0142159X.2018.1497149

Meo, A. I. (2010). Picturing students' habitus: The advantages and limitations of photo-elicitation interviewing in a qualitative study in the city of Buenos Aires. *International Journal of Qualitative Methods, 9*(2), 149–171. https://doi.org/10.1177/160940691000900203

Milasan, L. H. (2023). "Mending fractured personalities": A photography-based cultural study of recovery from mental distress in Romania. *Transcultural Psychiatry, 60*(2), 226–243. https://doi.org/10.1177/13634615221119373

Mortensen, M., & McCrow-Young, A. (2022). *Social media images and conflicts*. Routledge

Nobles, A. L., Leas, E. C., Noar, S., Dredze, M., Latkin, C. A., Strathdee, S. A., & Ayers, J. W. (2020). Automated image analysis of Instagram posts: Implications for risk perception and communication in public health using a case study of #HIV. *PLoS ONE, 15*(5), 1–11. https://doi.org/10.1371/journal.pone.0231155

Oliveira, L. M., Pilecco, K. de Souza, D. F., de Oliveira, C. A., & Zanatta, F. B. (2022). Main uses of Instagram in oral health research: A scoping review. *Health Policy and Technology, 11*(1), 1–10. https://doi.org/10.1016/j.hlpt.2022.100605

Palibroda, B., Krieg, B., Murdock, L., & Havelock, J. (2009). *A practical guide to photovoice: Sharing pictures, telling stories and changing communities*. https://rpay.link/guide/pdf20.pdf

Park, C. M., Han, S. J., Lee, J. H., Lim, J., Moon, S. D., Moon, H., Lee, S-Y., Kim, H., Jang, I-Y., & Jung, H-W. (2022). A focus group interview with health professionals: Establishing efficient transition care plan for older adult patients in Korea. *BMC Health Services Research, 22*(1), 1–10. https://doi.org/10.1186/s12913-022-07802-z

Reid, K., Elliot, D., Witayarat, N., & Wilson-Smith, K. (2018, October 17–19). *Reflecting on the use of photo-elicitation methods in IPA research. Enhancing the interpretative lens and re-balancing power back to the participant. A review of published studies*. World Conference on Qualitative Research, Lisbon, Portugal, pp. 108–109.

Tausch, A. P., & Menold, N. (2016). Methodological aspects of focus groups in health research: Results of qualitative interviews with focus group moderators. *Global Qualitative Nursing Research, 3*(1), 1–12. https://doi.org/10.1177/2333393616630466

Tricas-Vidal, H. J., Vidal-Peracho, M. C., Lucha-López, M. O., Hidalgo-García, C., Lucha-López, A. C., Monti-Ballano, S., Corral-de Toro, J., Márquez-Gonzalvo, S., Tricás-Moreno, J. M. (2022). Nutrition-related content on Instagram in the United States of America: Analytical cross-sectional study. *Foods, 11*(2), 1–13. https://doi.org/10.3390/foods11020239

Walstra, V. (2020). Picturing the group: Combining photo-elicitation and focus group methods. *Anthrovision, 8*(1), 1–23. https://doi.org/10.4000/anthrovision.6790

Wang, C. C. (1999). Photovoice: A participatory action research strategy applied to women's health. *Journal of Women's Health, 8*(2), 185–192. https://doi.org/10.1089/jwh.1999.8.185

Further reading

Brown, N. (2024). *Photovoice reimagined (creative research methods in Practice)*. Policy Press.

Edmondson, A. J., Borthwick, R., Hughes, E., & Lucock, M. (2022). Using photovoice to understand and improve healthy lifestyles of people diagnosed with serious mental illness. *Journal of Psychiatric and Mental Health Nursing, 29*(5), 676–687. https://doi.org/10.1111/jpm.12863

Milasan, L. H. (2022). Photo-elicitation: Unleashing imagery in healthcare research. In P. Ali, J. McGarry, & K. Hinsliff-Smith (Eds.), *Arts based health care research: A multidisciplinary perspective* (pp. 51–67). Springer International Publishing. https://doi.org/10.1007/978-3-030-94423-0_5

5

ANALYSIS AND INTERPRETATION OF PHOTOGRAPHS

5.1 The 5Cs of visual analysis

Analysing photographs, regardless of their source, for example, participant-generated, taken by the research team, or sourced from the Internet, is a crucial step in evaluating content and understanding the meanings attributed to the visual material by research participants. The volume of visual data generated through photographic interviews or focus groups can be overwhelming. Its analysis may require as much time and interpretative depth as the exploration of the verbal contributions of research participants to ensure a balanced and rigorous interpretation. Given the diversity of approaches in visual research shaped by disciplinary perspectives from anthropology, sociology, healthcare, psychology, and beyond, there is a clear need for a consistent and transparent analytical framework.

This chapter introduces the 5Cs of visual analysis – Content, Context, Composition, Connection, and Chronology – I advance here as a structured and memorable approach to guide researchers through the interpretive process. Each of these dimensions offers a distinct yet interrelated lens for examining images, enabling a more systematic and reflective engagement with visual data. By applying the 5Cs framework (summarised in Table 5.1), researchers can enhance the clarity, depth, and reporting of their visual analyses across diverse research settings.

5.1.1 Content

Content refers to the tangible and visible elements within a photograph such as people, animals, objects, landscapes, settings, and visual symbols. It encompasses both concrete, real-world features and metaphorical representations, particularly when meaning is encoded through visual metaphors.

Visual metaphors, illustrated in Figure 5.1, play a crucial role in healthcare research, particularly when exploring complex, sensitive, or abstract phenomena. Visual metaphors help translate intangible experiences such as pain, trauma, recovery, or emotional states into concrete, relatable imagery. This is especially valuable in qualitative research, where participants may struggle to articulate their experiences verbally.

DOI: 10.4324/9781003537540-6

TABLE 5.1 The 5Cs framework with prompts to deepen the analysis of photographs in a structured and reflective manner

Content What is in the image?	What objects, people, or elements are visible in the photograph? Are there any symbols or visual motifs present? What do they represent? Are there any recurring themes or patterns in the content? Is there anything missing from the picture?
Context What surrounds the image?	Where was the photograph taken? How does this influence its meaning? Who created the image, and for what purpose? What historical, social, or cultural factors might affect the interpretation of the image? How does the intended audience shape the message or impact of the image?
Composition How is the image composed?	How are elements positioned within the photograph? What draws the viewer's attention? What role do colour, light, and shadow play in shaping the image's tone or focus? Are there any lines, shapes, or textures that guide the viewer's eye? What is their meaning? What do the framing and perspective (e.g., close-up, wide shot) say about the photograph?
Connection How does the photograph relate to the research participant, the viewer (i.e., the researcher or broader audience), and the research topic?	What emotions or ideas does the photograph evoke in the research participants/viewer? How does the image connect to the personal experiences of the research participant or the broader cultural understanding of its audience? What broader themes, issues, or narratives does the photograph relate to? Does the photograph provoke action, thought, or change? If so, how?
Chronology What is the temporal dimension of the image?	When was the photograph taken? What moment in time does the image capture? Is it a decisive moment, a staged scene, or part of a sequence? How does the image relate to events before or after it was taken? How does the passage of time affect the interpretation or relevance of the image today? Are there visible signs of time (e.g., ageing, decay, growth, change) within the image itself?

While symbolic interpretation is often prioritised in visual analysis, the examination of concrete elements remains equally important. A facial expression, a natural landscape, or an everyday object can carry profound meaning, especially when such significance is explicitly articulated by the research participant.

In a photo-elicitation interview I conducted (Milasan, 2023), I initially felt a sense of disappointment when a participant did not elaborate on visual metaphors, as others had. However, this was simply because no metaphors were intended. The road depicted in their photograph (Figure 5.2) was not a symbolic journey toward light, punctuated by shadows representing life's challenges, as I envisaged. It was, quite literally, an alleyway leading to the community centre where the participant found companionship, peer support, and meaningful activities. This experience prompted critical reflection on my own interpretive tendencies potentially leading to bias,

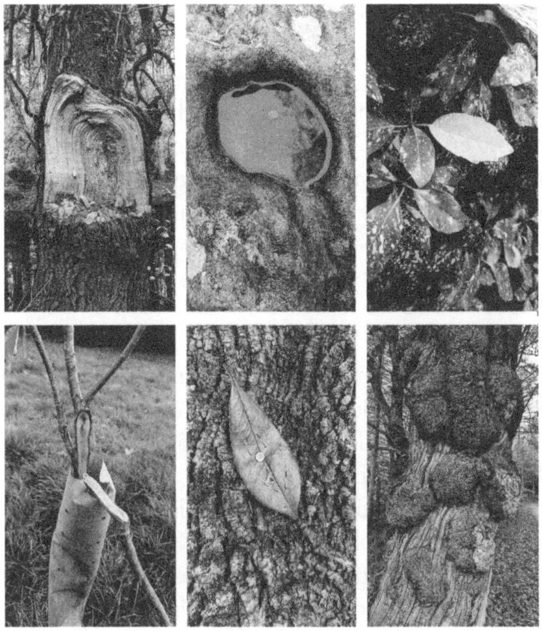

FIGURE 5.1 Nature-inspired metaphors of health and illness – “Excision” (top-left); “Kidney stones” (top-middle); “Vitiligo” (top-right); “Fracture” (bottom-left); “Transplant” (bottom-middle); “Moles” (bottom-right)

Source: photographs by the Author

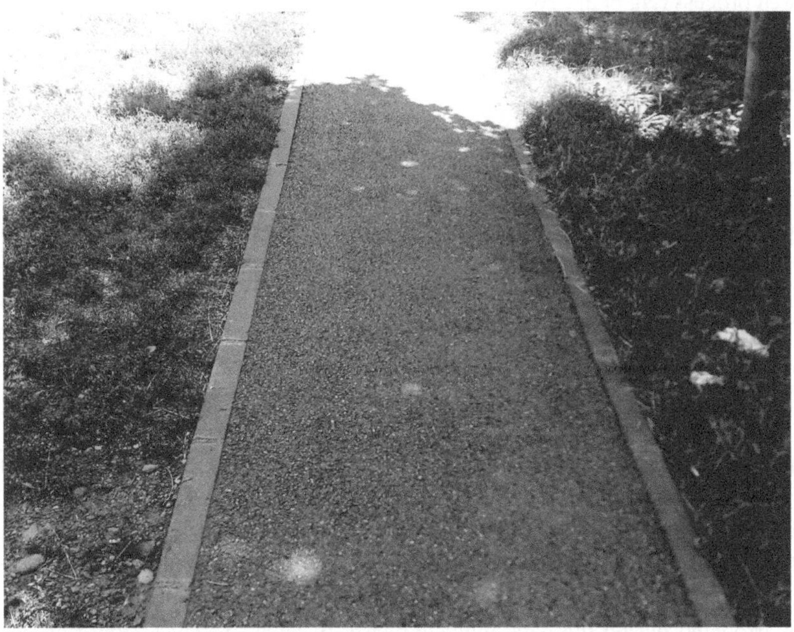

FIGURE 5.2 “My road to recovery”

Source: photograph by Mihai

and reminded me to prioritise participants' perspectives over my inclination to search for hidden or symbolic meanings.

Also important in analysing content is the need to immerse oneself in the image and consider not only what participants chose to include but also what they omitted. Absences can be just as revealing as presences, prompting further inquiry into the participant's intentions. In this sense, the process of analysing content resembles a jigsaw puzzle with each detail contributing to a broader narrative or message that gradually unfolds through careful observation and interpretation.

5.1.2 Context

Context explores the broader circumstances surrounding the creation and interpretation of a photograph. This includes the time, place, and cultural environment in which it was produced, as well as the creator's intentions. Without context, a photograph may lose much of its depth and significance. Similarly, removing a photograph from its context and stripping away background information can compromise the validity of the analysis and undermine the overall methodological and interpretative value of the study.

Such issues may lead to misinterpreting the photograph's message by ignoring socio-political, cultural, historical, or situational factors, oversimplifying its meaning, reinforcing researcher bias by projecting personal assumptions, and failing to connect the image to broader themes hidden in its contextual background.

Moreover, employing photographs without acknowledging their full context may raise ethical concerns. Participants may feel that their experiences have been misrepresented or reduced to narratives that fail to reflect their lived realities. This concern is especially pertinent in participatory research methodologies such as photovoice, where participants' perspectives are central to the research process (Ng et al., 2024).

5.1.3 Composition

Composition or the way visual elements are consciously or subconsciously arranged in a photograph is not merely about aesthetic appeal; it plays a critical role in shaping how meaning is constructed and communicated through an image. Composition involves the deliberate or intuitive structuring of visual elements such as space, balance, symmetry, perspective, light, shadow, and framing. These elements guide the viewer's eye, establish focal points, and influence emotional and cognitive responses. For instance, a photograph with a central subject framed symmetrically may evoke a sense of stability, as exemplified in Figure 5.3. Similarly, an off-centre composition might suggest movement, tension, or spontaneity. The use of light and shadow can dramatically alter the mood of an image highlighting certain features while obscuring others, thereby shaping interpretation (Figure 5.4).

Additional compositional features such as colour, exposure, shape, rhythm, and depth of field also contribute to the visual narrative. Colour can carry symbolic meaning or evoke emotional responses. For example, a participant I worked with in a photo-elicitation study associated the colour red with trauma and deliberately excluded this colour from her photographs. Similarly, depth of field or using the zoom feature can draw attention to specific elements that can be further interrogated during the data analysis phase. In many instances, these choices are not neutral – they reflect perspectives, priorities, and sometimes unconscious biases.

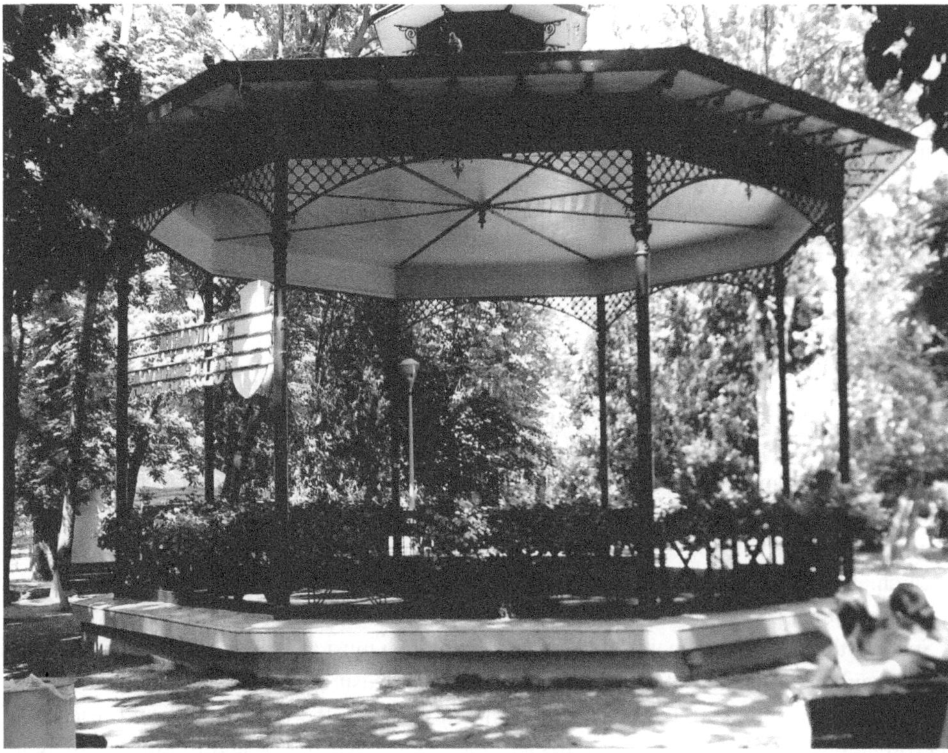

FIGURE 5.3 "Symmetry is a reflection of searching for stability; an attempt to feel grounded amidst uncertainty"

Source: photograph by Mihai

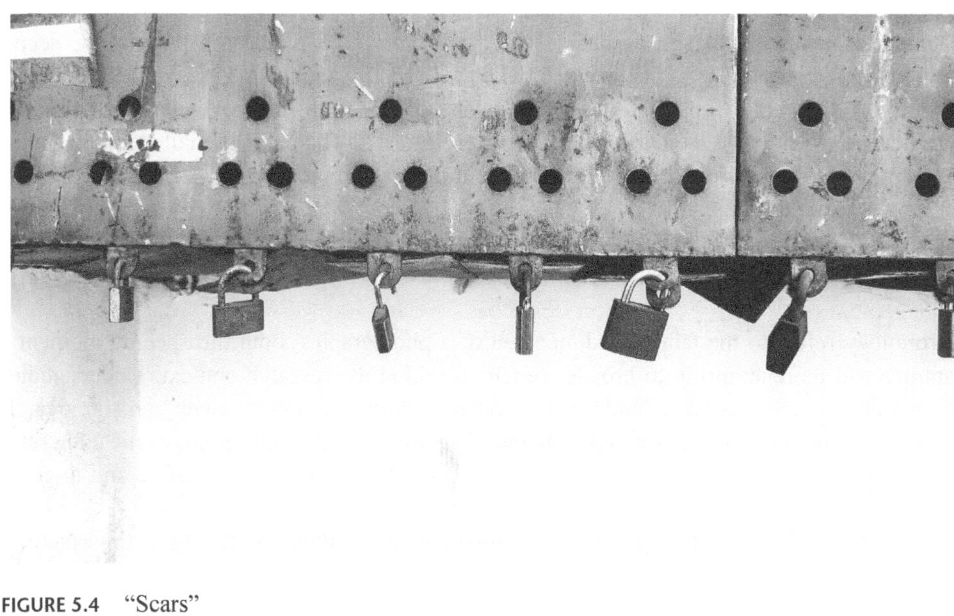

FIGURE 5.4 "Scars"

Source: photograph by Laura

In the context of visual data analysis, composition should be examined not for its artistic merit alone, but for how it contributes to the message, mood, and meaning of the image. A photograph's composition can reveal how participants frame their experiences, what they choose to emphasise or obscure, and how they position themselves in relation to the subject matter. For example, the photograph in Figure 5.4 can be interpreted as a visual metaphor for emotional healing: the top half reveals scars and traumas from the past – some still open, others closed, resolved – while the bottom half, with its white hues, suggests a calmer state of mind experienced by the individual in the present in spite of all the burden of the past.

5.1.4 Connections

Connections embedded within a photograph can be analysed on at least three levels.

First, it is critical to understand how research participants relate emotionally, intellectually, or culturally to the images they produced or were provided with. Thoughts and feelings are central to personal experience; therefore, it is challenging to capture participants' unique perspectives and voices without considering their connection to the photograph. This dimension reveals the power of an image to inspire thought, dialogue, and action – one of the core principles of photography-based research. Exploring participants' connections to the image ensures that the analysis remains grounded in their perspective and is not misappropriated to support unintended narratives.

Second, the researcher's connection to the photograph must also be critically examined. This helps avoid the projection of personal assumptions and ensures that interpretations are aligned with the participant's narrative. Any misalignment between the participant's and researcher's interpretations should be carefully reflected upon, and strategies to address these differences should be identified and implemented to minimise researcher bias.

Third, researchers must clarify how each photograph relates to the research question before drawing conclusions based on its content, context, or composition. Establishing this connection situates the image within a broader analytical framework, linking it to key themes, questions, or hypotheses relevant to the study.

In one instance, I was surprised to discover, together with a research participant, deeper meanings and connections to the research topic than initially anticipated. A series of seemingly repetitive photographs of natural landscapes I was inclined to dismiss, eventually revealed the significance of nature in the participant's recovery process. This insight challenged my initial assumption that the participant had deviated from the research topic and was using the camera for recreational purposes.

5.1.5 Chronology

Chronology refers to the temporal dimension of a photograph – both the specific moment it captures and its relationship to broader timelines within the research context. Understanding when a photograph was taken, and what preceded or followed that moment, can significantly influence its interpretation. A single image may freeze a fleeting instance, but its meaning often unfolds across time, shaped by events, memories, or changes that occur before and after the captured moment.

In visual research, analysing chronology involves more than identifying a timestamp; it requires situating the image within a narrative arc. This includes considering whether the photograph represents a beginning, a turning point, or a resolution in the participant's experience. For example, a photograph of an empty hospital corridor may carry different meanings depending on whether it was taken at the start of a treatment journey, during a moment of isolation, or after discharge. These temporal associations can reveal emotional trajectories, shifts in identity, or evolving relationships with place and self.

Chronology also plays a role in how photographs are sequenced and discussed during data collection. In photo-elicitation or photovoice interviews, the order in which images are presented or recalled can reflect the participant's sense of time, memory, and significance. Researchers must remain attentive to these cues, as they can offer insights into how participants construct meaning over time.

Chronology is particularly vital in narrative research, where the sequencing of events and the unfolding of personal stories are central to meaning-making. Photographs can serve as narrative anchors – visual cues that help participants recall, structure, and communicate their experiences over time. When analysed chronologically, images can reveal patterns of change, continuity, or disruption that might otherwise remain hidden. This temporal layering advances the narrative and allows researchers to trace how meaning develops across different phases of a participant's journey.

It can be noted that the 5Cs progress from descriptive, for example, looking at the image more objectively and taking in its details, to interpretive that is, drawing subjective meanings through reflection and critical interrogation of the image. Although presented separately, the 5Cs are interlinked. For example, omitting the context or background information of a photograph may have implications for the depth of reflective responses.

5.2 Coding and corroborating visual and textual data

Qualitative healthcare research has traditionally focused on textual data. However, shifts in research practices have expanded qualitative coding to include other media such as photographs, artwork, and videography. As a result, qualitative software such as NVivo®, MAXQDA®, QDA Miner®, and ATLAS.ti® now accommodate visual data analysis, providing tools specifically designed for this purpose. Due to copyright restrictions, this section does not provide examples of software tool applications widely available through online resources that are easily accessible to researchers. Instead, key principles of image coding will be outlined to support visual data analysis, whether conducted manually or adapted for use with qualitative analysis software.

Regardless of the method used, coding is a crucial step in visual data analysis, allowing the researcher to deconstruct the dataset into meaningful units of analysis. These units are then reconstructed and triangulated with textual data to identify themes and narratives relevant to answering the research question guiding the study (Rose, 2022).

First of all, it is important to ensure that photographs from a series of photo-elicitation interviews or photography workshops conducted by the researcher are labelled with unique identifiers. This step will make it easier for researchers to keep track of the photographs and their associated codes in a spreadsheet or a database, along with their links to textual data. The process of linking images and text in qualitative research is known as data triangulation, a technique that is known to contribute to enhancing the rigour of the research by minimising bias (Carter et al., 2014). This is because the data analysis starts with participants' interpretations instead of relying on the researcher's decontextualised analysis of photographs.

After a framework to organise the photographs was established by the researcher, the next task consists of familiarisation with the visual data. This step consists of reviewing the photographs and transcripts multiple times, preferably by taking notes on initial impressions, thoughts, and emotional tones. By doing so, the researcher begins to get immersed not only in the content and meaning of the photographs but also in the context in which the photographs were taken and presented (see the 5Cs approach explained in the previous section).

As with textual analysis, visual data can be coded using either deductive or inductive approaches. *Deductive* or *a priori coding* relies on pre-established categories often derived from previous research, which are applied to the data as analysis progresses. In contrast, *inductive coding* involves reviewing data to identify codes, patterns, and themes that are identified organically rather than being predetermined. Bingham (2023) provides a comprehensive description of both approaches, which are often combined in a hybrid strategy (Fereday & Muir-Cochrane, 2006).

While deductive coding may offer consistency and structure, the decision to use this approach must consider its potential limitations. A common criticism of deductive coding is that it may introduce bias by relying on predetermined codes, potentially leading researchers to overlook new or unexpected themes. This makes it less suitable for exploratory research, where an inductive strategy is often preferred (Morse & Mitcham, 2002).

However, inductive coding is not without its challenges. For instance, achieving inter-coder reliability (i.e., consistency between different coders) can be difficult when coding categories are not predefined, which may affect the rigour of the study, particularly for less experienced researchers. Moreover, inductive coding requires a careful balance between deep immersion in the data and maintaining focus on research aims, making it a time-intensive process (Morse & Mitcham, 2002).

Ultimately, the choice of coding approach depends on the research objectives. For example, deductive coding may be more appropriate for testing theoretical frameworks, while inductive coding is better suited for exploring complex phenomena and lived experiences. Regardless of the approach, it is essential for researchers to be transparent about their coding strategy when reporting findings.

Another important consideration is the level of coding, which ranges from descriptive to interpretative. When analysing photographs, descriptive coding involves noting observable details such as objects, people, settings, composition, spatial arrangement, and focal points. At the interpretative level, the researcher shifts focus to underlying meanings and narratives within the broader context. This level is particularly important for decoding visual metaphors and symbols, drawing on participants' own interpretations rather than relying on the researcher's assumptions.

By repeating this process across participants, for example, in photo-elicitation interviews, the researcher can begin to identify patterns and refine the links between textual codes and visual elements. This stage corresponds to thematic coding, where photographs and transcript excerpts are grouped into overarching themes. However, the researcher's analytical journey is rarely linear. On the contrary, it typically involves ongoing revisiting of photographs and accompanying text, along with iterative refinement of the coding framework and themes that are identified. When multiple researchers are involved, this iterative process includes collaborative review of preliminary codes to validate interpretations and consider alternative perspectives.

The process of deconstructing a photograph into key visual elements that guide photo-elicited conversations – from descriptive observations to deeper symbolic meanings – is illustrated in Figure 5.5. For context, the photograph was taken by Robert (pseudonym), a participant involved in a series of weekly workshops as part of a cultural study of recovery from mental

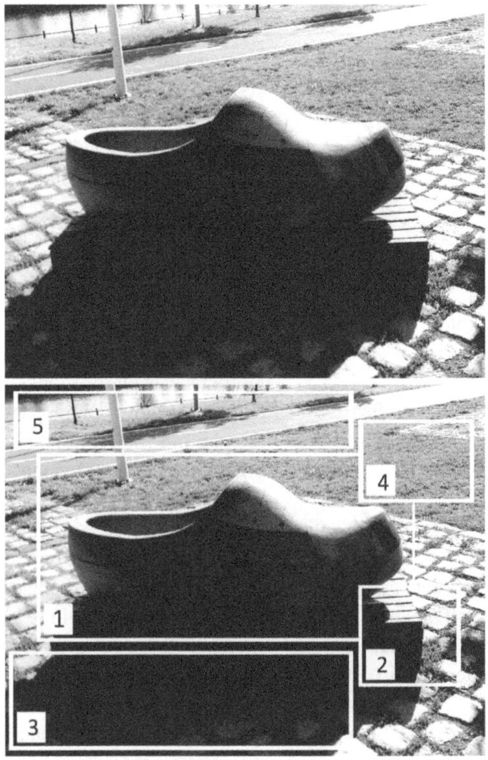

FIGURE 5.5 Deconstructing a photograph into its main visual elements

Source: photograph by Robert

distress (Milasan, 2023). The visual analysis of this photograph is complemented by Table 5.2 that integrates the visual elements with the participant's verbal contributions to support the process of meaning-making, guided by the 5Cs technique, and the list of codes in Table 5.3. This process reiterates the importance of analysing visual and verbal (or textual) data as complementary sources of knowledge. It is nearly impossible to derive meaning solely from visual elements without making interpretive assumptions. Conversely, certain meanings and narratives may be difficult to construct without visual elements, which often evoke subconscious thoughts, emotions, and memories that enrich the data.

Analysing visual content in photographs can be approached through a *hermeneutic* lens – a theoretical and interpretive framework grounded in philosophical traditions, particularly the work of Hans-Georg Gadamer and Paul Ricoeur. Hermeneutics emphasises the dialogical and context-dependent nature of meaning-making, recognising that interpretation is shaped by the interplay between the viewer and the image, each bringing their own histories, perspectives, and preconceptions. Rather than seeking fixed or universal meanings, hermeneutic analysis acknowledges that meaning is dynamic and co-constructed (Alsaigh & Coyne, 2021). This perspective aligns closely with participatory research principles, as it encourages reflexive engagement with participants' interpretations and positions data analysis as a collaborative process. In visual research, a hermeneutic approach deepens understanding by attending not only to what is

TABLE 5.2 Excerpts from a photo-elicitation interview guided by the 5Cs technique

Content What objects, people, or elements are visible in the photograph?	"There are many things going on in this photograph, starting with the wooden clog [1]. I believe it's some sort of artwork; I don't know how it ended there in the park, but I liked it and I decided to take a photo of it. And there is the wooden base [2], the pavement or cobblestones [3], the grass [4], and a road or, well, a bike lane [5], and the river in the background, mostly lines and patterns".
Context When and where was the photograph taken?	"The picture was taken during one of my long walks in a nearby park when I came across this unusual object that stood out from me".
Composition How are elements positioned within the photograph? What draws the viewer's attention?	"My focus was on the wooden clog that is obviously the star of the show [laughs] so I placed it at the centre of the photo. I tried to frame it in a way that reflects how big and heavy it is. I managed to include a road [5] in the photo that I thought it works well with the wooden clog".
Connections How does the research participant connect with the photograph on an emotional and narrative level? What meanings lie behind the elements in the photograph?	"I like walking in the park and nature, in general. And this wooden clog was an accurate representation of this idea. I found it a little weird and quirky, like me [laughs]! What I was trying to say in this picture is that walking and keeping active is an important thing to do for my mental health. One step at the time [laughs]". "I was talking about the road to recovery that sometimes does not seem to go anywhere like this heavy wooden clog fixed on that pallet. It makes me think about the burden of my mental illness, how difficult it is sometimes to move on with my life. You need more people to make a move with this clog [laughs]. Like in real life, really. You can't get better in isolation. At the same time, it could also represent stability, which is equally important in recovery." "Imagine if we [people with mental health difficulties] would wear wooden clogs like this one, and all the noise we would make in society marching around and drawing some attention to the stigma around mental illness. It would definitely cause a stir, or even an earthquake [laughs]!"
Chronology When was the photograph taken, and how does its timing influence the way the participant understands or relates to it at this point in time?	"This photo was taken early in my recovery, when I was still unsure about everything. Looking back now, I see it differently – it's not just a weird object in the park anymore. It is the beginning of something. At the time, I didn't realise how much that walk meant, but now I do. It was the first step, literally and metaphorically".

TABLE 5.3 List of codes based on the interpretation of visual and textual contributions captured in Figure 5.5 and Table 5.2

Wooden clog	Unusual object/Quirky (personality) Heavy/Burden Walking/Physical activity/Steps/Journey Marching/Anti-Stigma activism
Wooden pallet	Support/Foundation/Stability
Pavement/cobblestones	Intricate texture/Pathway/Road to recovery
Grass	Nature/Grounding/Calm
Road or bike lane	Direction/Journey
River in background	Flow/Nature
Lines and patterns	Visual rhythm/Structure/Complexity

depicted in the image but also to how participants relate to and reflect upon the visual material they produce or select, thereby enriching both the interpretive depth and ethical integrity of the research.

Alongside hermeneutics, *iconography* offers another valuable method for analysing visual data, particularly in research involving participant-generated imagery. Iconographic analysis involves systematic identification, description, and interpretation of visual content, aiming to uncover both literal (denotative) and symbolic (connotative) meanings embedded in images. These meanings are often situated within specific cultural, historical, or social contexts, making iconography especially useful for exploring how visual elements communicate shared or contested understandings. Drawing on Erwin Panofsky's (1955) influential framework, iconographic analysis typically unfolds across three levels: 1. pre-iconographic description or identification of basic visual elements without interpretation; 2. iconographic analysis focused on interpreting the conventional meanings of these elements; and 3. iconological interpretation involving a deeper exploration of cultural, historical, or ideological meanings, often requiring contextual knowledge.

While iconography offers a structured and insightful method for interpreting visual data, it also presents limitations, particularly when analysis is conducted solely by researchers without involving participants. In such cases, interpretations may reflect the researchers' cultural assumptions or theoretical biases, potentially overlooking or misrepresenting the meanings intended by participants. The next section elaborates on the importance of including participants in the data analysis process, highlighting how collaborative interpretation not only enhances the validity and contextual relevance of findings but also aligns with ethical commitments to equity, representation, and shared ownership of knowledge.

5.3 The role of participants in analysing photographic data

In a systematic review focused on photography-based methods in mental health recovery research (Milasan et al., 2020), I highlighted the issue of limited participant involvement in analysing photographs as research data. Similar critiques have emerged across other areas of healthcare, where researchers are traditionally regarded as the primary holders of analytical expertise (Locock et al., 2019). However, the notion of "expertise" has been increasingly challenged by the rise of participatory research in healthcare, which places greater emphasis on involving participants beyond the data collection stage.

These approaches often culminate in co-production, where shared power and decision-making, including during data analysis, are central to ensuring an inclusive, transparent, and democratic research process. Ride (2015), reflecting on their experience of involving participants in data analysis, concluded that while the process can be time- and resource-consuming (including research training for participants), it effectively addresses the traditional imbalance of power between researchers and participants.

Moreover, involving participants in data analysis creates opportunities for new interpretations and insights. This redistribution of analytical responsibility is equitable, recognising participants' contributions to knowledge production and enabling them to influence how findings are presented and represented. While some may argue that engaging participants in data analysis is impractical due to a lack of technical expertise, emerging participatory and collaborative frameworks challenge this notion. These approaches aim to "integrate inclusive and transparent data interpretation into the research cycle, and support the identification of relevant and contextually-informed research findings" (Scott-Barrett et al., 2023, p. 1). Such frameworks emphasise capacity-building through training, ensuring that participants or co-researchers are effectively equipped to contribute meaningfully.

The rationale for participant involvement is grounded in various theoretical perspectives with potential for (democratising etc.) for democratising the research process. These range from constructivist and interpretivist paradigms, which promote socially constructed and context-dependent knowledge (van der Walt, 2020), to critical theories that support participant involvement as a means of challenging traditional power dynamics in knowledge production (Kemmis, 2008). Nonetheless, the literature remains ambiguous about the practical steps required to transition from a researcher-led model to one that genuinely incorporates participants in shaping analytical outcomes. However, several examples of good practice exist and offer replicable models for inclusive data analysis, such as Participatory Research Oxford (PROX) and the Participatory Action Research (PAR) Toolkit developed by researchers at the University of Reading, included in the list of further reading at the end of this chapter.

An example of good practice in qualitative research is employing member checking, that is, a process that typically occurs at the end of a study, allowing researchers to address any misunderstandings or misinterpretations in collaboration with research participants. However, some scholars advocate for participant involvement in data analysis throughout the research process, not only at the conclusion of the study, to enhance reflexivity (Ride, 2015). This is particularly relevant when working with participants from disadvantaged, exploited, or oppressed backgrounds, whose voices are equally important in both data collection and analysis. This is to ensure that their perspectives are accurately represented and not distorted by researcher bias or political agendas.

This aspect is critical in healthcare research, where numerous studies involve vulnerable populations whose perspectives have historically been muted due to intersecting social, political, and cultural factors. Fundamentally, it involves shifting from conducting research on passive "subjects" to actively collaborating with participants in the co-production of knowledge. Within this process, both the academic expertise of researchers and the experiential knowledge of participants, such as those with lived experience of physical and/or mental health conditions, are recognised. Similarly, it entails transforming research from an instrument of power that may perpetuate inequities or serve hidden agendas into a platform for amplifying participant voices and generating knowledge that is directly relevant to those involved.

Creating opportunities for decision-making at all stages of research should be recognised as a right of research participants, rather than a privilege granted by researchers and embedded within academic discourse. Photography, like other visual media, serves as an effective form of expression that can make participant involvement in data analysis more accessible, particularly for individuals with limited literacy skills, compared to more text-heavy or technical research methods. Visual elements, in this context, offer alternative avenues for participants to contribute not only to data generation but also to its critical analysis from their own perspectives, thereby enhancing the validity of the findings and ensuring they are representative of participants' lived experiences.

This growing emphasis on inclusive data analysis reflects a broader shift within healthcare towards participatory and person-centred approaches. Just as patients are increasingly recognised as active partners in their own care, through shared decision-making, co-design of services, and patient-led advocacy, research participants are being acknowledged as co-creators of knowledge. This alignment underscores a fundamental transformation in both practice and research from hierarchical, expert-driven models to collaborative frameworks that value lived experience, promote equity, and enhance the relevance and impact of research outcomes.

Conclusion

Analysing and interpreting photographs in healthcare research is not a purely technical exercise – it is a deeply interpretive process that demands methodological rigour and reflexivity. The 5Cs framework (Content, Context, Composition, Connection, Chronology) advanced in this chapter offers a structured approach for addressing the challenges of visual data, moving from descriptive observation to critical interpretation. However, it is important to remember that photographs rarely speak in isolation; their meanings emerge through dialogue with participants and triangulation with textual data. Involving participants in the analytical process is not only an ethical imperative but also a methodological strength, ensuring that interpretations remain grounded in their lived experience rather than researcher assumptions.

Knowledge check

1. What are the potential implications of analysing visual and textual data from a photo-elicitation interview separately rather than an integrated dataset?
2. What challenges might arise when involving research participants in the analysis of data generated through photography workshops in which they actively participated?

References

Alsaigh, R., & Coyne, I. (2021). Doing a hermeneutic phenomenology research underpinned by Gadamer's philosophy: A framework to facilitate data analysis. *International Journal of Qualitative Methods, 20*(1), 1–10. https://doi.org/10.1177/16094069211047820

Bingham, A. J. (2023). From data management to actionable findings: A five-phase process of qualitative data analysis. *International Journal of Qualitative Methods, 22*(1), 1–11. https://doi.org/10.1177/16094069231183620

Carter, N., Bryant-Lukosius, D., DiCenso, A., Blythe, J., & Neville, A. J. (2014). The use of triangulation in qualitative research. *Oncology Nursing Forum, 41*(5), 545–547. https://doi.org/10.1188/14.ONF.545-547

Fereday, J., & Muir-Cochrane, E. (2006). Demonstrating rigor using thematic analysis: A hybrid approach of inductive and deductive coding and theme development. *International Journal of Qualitative Methods, 5*(1), 80–92. https://doi.org/10.1177/160940690600500107

Kemmis, S. (2008). Critical theory and participatory action research. In P. Reason & H. Bradbury (Eds.), *Critical theory and participatory action research* (2nd ed., pp. 121–138). SAGE Publications Ltd. https://doi.org/10.4135/9781848607934.n14

Locock, L., Kirkpatrick, S., Brading, L., Sturmey, G., Cornwell, J., Churchill, N., & Robert, G. (2019). Involving service users in the qualitative analysis of patient narratives to support healthcare quality improvement. *Research Involvement & Engagement, 5*(1), 1–11. https://doi.org/10.1186/s40900-018-0133-z

Milasan, L. H. (2023). "Mending fractured personalities": A photography-based cultural study of recovery from mental distress in Romania. *Transcultural Psychiatry, 60*(2), 226–243. https://doi.org/10.1177/13634615221119373

Milasan, L. H., Bingley, A. F., & Fisher, N. R. (2020). The big picture of recovery: A systematic review on the evidence of photography-based methods in researching recovery from mental distress. *Arts & Health, 14*(2), 165–185. https://doi.org/10.1080/17533015.2020.1855453

Morse, J. M., & Mitcham, C. (2002). Exploring qualitatively-derived concepts: Inductive – deductive pitfalls. *International Journal of Qualitative Methods, 1*(4), 28–35. https://doi.org/10.1177/160940690200100404

Ng, C. G., Ting, S. Q., Saifi, R. A., & Kamarulzaman, A. B. (2024). Ethical issues in photovoice studies involving key populations: A scoping review. *Asian Bioethics Review, 16*(1), 109–129. https://doi.org/10.1007/s41649-023-00264-3

Panofsky, E. (1955). Iconography and iconology: An introduction to the study of renaissance art. In E. Panofsky (Ed.), *Meaning in the visual arts: Papers in and on art history* (pp. 26–54). Doubleday.

Ride, A. (2015). Involving participants in data analysis. In D. Bretherton & S. Law (Eds.), *Methodologies in peace psychology* (pp. 129–221). Springer. https://doi.org/10.1007/978-3-319-18395-4_10

Rose, G. (2022). *Visual methodologies. An introduction to researching with visual materials*. University of Oxford.

Scott-Barrett, J., Marshall-Brown, A., Livingstone-Banks, M., Chrisinger, B., Scher, B., & Hickman, M. (2023). *Participatory research: Researcher insights*. University of Oxford. https://www.ox.ac.uk/research/using-research-engage/public-engagement/participatory-research

van der Walt, J. (2020). Interpretivism-constructivism as a research method in the humanities and social sciences – more to it than meets the eye. *International Journal of Philosophy and Theology, 8*(1), 59–68. https://doi.org/10.15640/ijpt.v8n1a5

Further reading

University of Oxford. (2023). *Participatory Research Oxford (PROX)*. https://www.ox.ac.uk/research/using-research-engage/public-engagement/participatory-research

University of Reading. (2023). *Participatory Action Research (PAR) toolkit*. https://research.reading.ac.uk/community-based-research/wp-content/uploads/sites/114/2023/06/PAR-Toolkit-v10.pdf

6

REPORTING AND DISSEMINATING FINDINGS

6.1 Guidelines for writing up photography-based research

This section draws upon my experience as a visual researcher and my role as a reviewer for journal articles focused on photography-based research. Through my journey as a published researcher, I have gained invaluable insights not only from fieldwork but also from the constructive feedback received on my submitted manuscripts. This feedback has significantly contributed to my professional development and advanced my academic writing. It also enabled me to provide informed and constructive critiques to other researchers in my capacity as a reviewer. The insights presented in this section are particularly focused on identifying and addressing gaps in photography-based published research, including both my own work and that of others. By addressing these gaps, healthcare researchers can significantly enhance the robustness of photography-based studies and improve the quality of reporting and manuscripts submitted for publication.

6.1.1 Rationale for employing photographic techniques in healthcare research

Despite the extensive body of literature that incorporates photographic techniques, the distinctive advantages of employing photography in healthcare research remain insufficiently recognised (Pasquali, 2020). Photography has been frequently utilised to enhance visibility and innovation in research, especially in our era marked by technological advancements. However, the underlying rationale for its use is often inadequately articulated (Achiam et al., 2025). It is imperative to elucidate the unique capacity of photographs to capture dimensions of health phenomena that may elude other research methodologies. This task is crucial for positioning photography as a research method that offers additional insights beyond those provided by traditional or conventional approaches. Normally, this information is provided in the introductory section of a journal publication.

For instance, in qualitative research, photographic techniques can significantly enhance the accuracy and depth of healthcare research findings (Cleland & MacLeod, 2021). Photographs can capture nuanced details and contextual elements that might be overlooked by other methods,

DOI: 10.4324/9781003537540-7

thereby providing a richer and more comprehensive understanding of the subject matter. The methodological rationale for employing photographic techniques can be substantiated through examples of research projects within healthcare and other disciplines that have successfully utilised these methods. Additionally, the theoretical compatibility between photographic techniques and specific research paradigms further underscores their value (Alves et al., 2021). For example, phenomenology, with its focus on lived experiences and subjective realities, aligns well with the visual and interpretive nature of photography, thereby reinforcing the methodological robustness of this approach (Sitvast & Springer, 2020).

Expanding on this, it is essential to consider how photographic techniques can be integrated into healthcare research to maximise their potential. This involves not only the careful selection and use of photographic equipment but also the development of solid analytical frameworks for interpreting visual data. By advancing a well-founded rationale for the use of photographic techniques, researchers can contribute to the broader acceptance and integration of visual methods in healthcare research, ultimately enriching the field with deeper and more nuanced insights.

6.1.2 Methodological considerations

The rationale for incorporating photography into the research design can significantly strengthen the methodological foundation of a study. A critical methodological consideration involves ensuring the reliability and validity of photographic data. For this reason, researchers must meticulously document the processes used to capture and analyse photographs, thereby establishing the credibility of visual data. Additionally, the choice of photography as a research method may influence the recruitment process, potentially introducing biases that need to be carefully examined and mitigated.

Within this context, reflexivity is an important part of the methodological report, in which researchers should critically reflect on their own biases, assumptions, and influence on the research process (Olmos-Vega et al., 2023). This is because the way a researcher frames, selects, and interprets photographs is inherently subjective. Including a positionality statement that addresses the researcher's relationship to photography, for example, whether they are trained in visual arts, and their assumptions about visual representation, adds transparency and depth. By critically reflecting on their photographic choices and acknowledging their influence, researchers can mitigate bias and enhance the trustworthiness of their findings. This includes discussing how images were selected, how participants were involved in interpreting them, and how visual data were integrated with other forms of data.

Ethical considerations are another important area to consider when reporting photographic research, encompassing issues such as informed consent, privacy, and copyright detailed in Chapter 7. Researchers must identify and address ethical challenges with diligence, ensuring that participants' rights and dignity are upheld. Addressing these challenges not only safeguards ethical standards but also contributes to the broader knowledge base by providing insights into the complexities of conducting ethical photographic research (Langmann & Pick, 2018). Discussing these difficulties and proposing solutions can guide future researchers in adopting more ethical practices in photography-based research. It is also important to focus on the legal frameworks that govern the use of photography in research, including copyright laws and regulations related to the use of images that may vary in different geographic contexts.

An underreported aspect is the training of researchers and participants in the effective use of photographic techniques. For example, cultural sensitivity, that is, ensuring respect for cultural norms and values, when using photographs as a research method in healthcare is often overlooked. Adequate training ensures that photographs are captured with the necessary technical proficiency and contextual sensitivity. Furthermore, providing detailed information about the photographic equipment, settings, and environmental conditions can help establish clear documentation protocols for capturing and analysing photographic data. This transparency is crucial for the reproducibility of research, as it allows other researchers to understand, replicate, and critically evaluate the photographic methods and conditions under which the data were generated (Davda & Pasquali, 2020).

Contributions of research participants might extend beyond mere data collection, particularly in participatory and co-production studies. For example, participants can play an active role in curating photographs and shaping the narrative of the research, thereby ensuring their perspectives and voices are accurately represented (Newransky et al., 2024). Involving participants in the data analysis process further enhances the methodological rigour of the project, fostering a collaborative and inclusive research environment.

Additionally, the use of advanced software tools for visual analysis, such as image recognition algorithms and qualitative data analysis software, needs to be disclosed. Researchers should explain how these tools enhanced the accuracy and efficiency of analysing photographic data. Alternatively, they should also consider how such tools might hinder participants' voice, potentially introducing interpretive bias or distancing the analysis from the participants' intended meanings, as suggested by Ntsobi et al. (2024).

By thoroughly exploring these methodological and ethical considerations, researchers can produce more robust and impactful findings. This comprehensive approach not only enhances the quality of the research but also promotes the integration of photographic techniques as a valuable tool in the researcher's methodological repertoire. Furthermore, such rigour and transparency can significantly increase the appeal of the research to academic publishers, who often prioritise studies that demonstrate methodological clarity, ethical integrity, and innovative approaches.

6.1.3 Writing up the findings

To effectively articulate the findings, researchers must thoroughly organise and present the photographic data in a clear and coherent manner. There is a prevalent tendency to present findings predominantly from the researchers' perspective, which can inadvertently introduce bias (Holm, 2014). Hence, the importance of considering a section on reflexivity and positionality, as previously mentioned, before delving into the presentation of research findings.

Researchers must immerse themselves deeply in the data and strive to write up the findings in a manner that authentically reflects the perspectives of research participants, ensuring their voices are prominently heard. For instance, it is often unclear what criteria researchers use to curate the photographs included in the findings and the extent of participants' input in this selection process, as highlighted by Richard and Lahman (2015). In some cases, photographs are completely omitted from the presentation of findings, which undermines the purpose of incorporating photographic methods and renders the findings incomplete.

When reporting their findings, researchers should structure the narrative around key themes and patterns identified through the exploration of photographic data, supported by textual data such as quotes from participants. This approach not only enhances the richness of the findings but also ensures that the visual and textual elements complement each other, providing a holistic understanding of the research outcomes. Trombeta and Cox (2022) introduced the Textual-Visual Thematic Analysis (TVTA) framework to guide the integrated analysis of visual and textual data in photography-based research. Their approach shows not only how findings are derived but also underscores the value of making the research process transparent, enabling audiences to learn from both the research insights and the methodological processes behind them.

By addressing these methodological considerations, researchers can produce a more balanced, transparent, and comprehensive presentation of their findings, thereby enhancing the credibility and impact of their photographic research. Furthermore, they can showcase methodological innovation and originality by using photography creatively as a stand-alone method or combined with other artistic endeavours.

6.1.4 Discussing the findings

Discussing the findings of photographic research is crucial for contextualising the results within the existing body of literature on the research topic and within the theoretical frameworks that underpin the study. A common pitfall in the discussion section is the excessive repetition of findings or, more problematically, the introduction of new findings that were not presented in the results section. Instead, the discussion should focus on comparing and contrasting the results with existing literature, highlighting how the findings align with, differ from, or extend current knowledge.

In addition to situating the findings within the broader academic discourse, it is important to address the limitations and advantages of using photographic methods in the study. This balanced discussion can provide valuable insights into the strengths and weaknesses of photographic techniques, informing both research and practice. By acknowledging these limitations, researchers can offer insights that could add to the credibility and transparency of their study.

Cross-disciplinary insights can be reflected upon in the discussion section, especially when photography is used in conjunction with arts and other forms of technology such as digital imaging, 3D or AI-generated imagery, and virtual or augmented reality (Cleland & MacLeod, 2021). This may lead to discussions regarding collaborative approaches between healthcare professionals and professionals from other fields, such as visual arts and media studies, to promote the use of photographic techniques and outputs.

The discussion should also explore the implications of the photographic findings for practice. In healthcare-related studies, for example, this might involve considering how visual data can inform clinical decision-making, enhance patient communication, or support trauma-informed care. Equally important, the discussion section should include recommendations for future research that could guide subsequent studies by suggesting new avenues for exploration and potential methodological improvements. By providing a comprehensive and reflective discussion, researchers can contribute to the ongoing development of photographic methods in research, ultimately advancing the field.

6.2 Ideas for presenting findings from photographic research in healthcare

6.2.1 Visual storytelling

Storytelling is a powerful tool in healthcare research and practice, offering unique ways to engage audiences on a deeply human level. By employing narrative frameworks, researchers can convey the experiences, perspectives, and emotions of patients, healthcare providers, and communities, making their findings more relatable, memorable, and impactful.

Visual storytelling through photographs, for example, photo-narratives, captures attention and makes complex healthcare issues such as HIV (Schrader et al., 2011), breast cancer (Gurrieri & Drenten, 2019), and multiple sclerosis (Bolaki, 2016) easier to understand. Photographic narratives are conducive to empathy, encouraging audiences to see the health phenomena through the eyes of those affected. This can lead to greater advocacy and support for healthcare initiatives as illustrated in Young et al.'s (2024) study in which digital storytelling was used to challenge stigmatising cultural and institutional narratives surrounding substance use.

Additionally, visual storytelling can bridge the gap between technical research and public understanding, translating jargon into accessible language, while promoting the voice of the research participants. This approach is increasingly used in health promotion initiatives, drawing on visual storytelling combining photographs with videos, voice-overs, drawing, and other creative approaches (Brooks et al., 2022). Ultimately, stories inspire action, motivating stakeholders and the public to engage with and support improvements in healthcare practices and outcomes. For this reason, visual storytelling is frequently used in participatory research aiming to create social impact and opportunities for change, particularly for marginalised populations like individuals with intellectual disabilities (Harris et al., 2022).

From a plethora of visual storytelling approaches, photo-diaries, photobooks, story boards, and collages are explored in depth in the following sections.

Photo-diaries

A photo-diary is a chronological collection of photographs that document daily life, events, or experiences over a period of time. Photographs are often accompanied by written or oral narratives that provide context and personal reflections. This method allows researchers to capture the lived experiences of individuals in a detailed and nuanced manner (Volpe, 2019). Participants are actively involved in documenting their experiences, which can lead to more authentic content that can strengthen the research impact. Photo-diaries provide longitudinal insights by allowing for the documentation of changes and developments over time, which is key in researching health conditions.

This approach is illustrated by Kuo et al. (2022), who used photo-diaries alongside focus groups to explore the needs of community-dwelling older adults with chronic diseases in Taiwan in the context of digital disease management. Participants documented their daily routines and health-related behaviours through photographs, which facilitated deeper reflection and discussion during focus groups. This method enabled researchers to uncover participants' lived experiences, preferences, and challenges, ultimately informing the design of more responsive and user-centred digital health interventions.

Photo-diaries can provide valuable knowledge on the progression of health conditions, the impact of interventions, and the adaptation of individuals to their circumstances. They are often used in researching healthcare providers who can share their experiences of delivering care, or involvement in community healthcare initiatives, for example. This can be valuable for promoting such initiatives and evaluating their impact. For example, Utomo et al. (2025) describe how team photo-diaries were used by researchers and field staff in Cambodia to document and reflect on their experiences during a community health census. The method not only facilitated data collection but also contributed to enhancing collaboration, reflexivity, and visibility of local knowledge and power dynamics in global health research.

To assist research participants to create effective photo-diaries, the purpose of the photo-diary should be clearly defined in line with the research aim. The researchers should also provide participants with clear instructions on how to take and select photographs, and discuss the types of moments and experiences to capture that are significant to their illness, health, or healthcare journey. However, the researchers should give participants some flexibility to encourage creativity by facilitating opportunities to document their experiences with a written or audio-recorded narrative or journal entry to accompany their photographs (Figure 6.1).

Photobooks

Photobooks are valuable tools for presenting photographic research in healthcare, sharing some similarities with photo-diaries. Photobooks can be defined as curated collections of photographs often organised around a specific theme or narrative, presented in a book format. They are designed to be visually appealing and impactful for the target audiences, and professionally produced, which makes them suitable for more formal presentations and publications (Parr & Badger, 2004).

The audiences for photobooks tend to be centred around stakeholders, policymakers, and the general public, for which reason advocacy and communication are key aspects of this approach. However, photobooks are often used in working with patients. For example, at the Royal Lancaster Infirmary in the UK, a staff member created a photobook filled with images of local landmarks to support patient well-being (NHS, 2021). The initiative was particularly aimed at

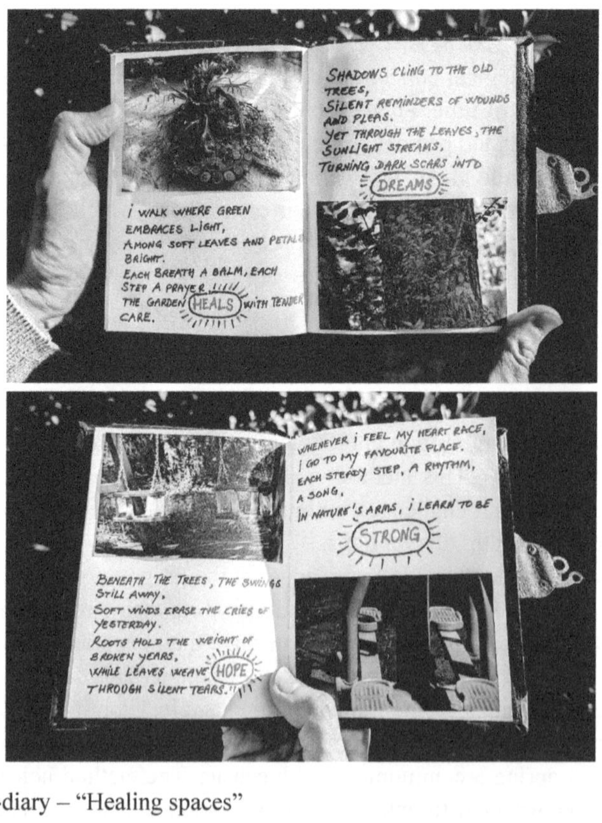

FIGURE 6.1 Photo-diary – "Healing spaces"

Source: photographs by Judit – top-right and bottom-left; Rodion – top-left; and Călin – bottom-right sparking conversation, evoking memories, and providing comfort – especially for patients living with dementia. The photobook served not only as a visual stimulus but also as a therapeutic tool to enhance patient experience and engagement during hospital stays.

Another innovative use of this technique is exemplified in Dodd et al.'s (2022) study, where an artist-produced photobook was used as an educational tool to support nurses and nursing students in learning about dementia. The photobook combined images and narratives to evoke emotional responses and stimulate reflection, helping participants to better understand the lived experiences of people with dementia. The study found that the photobook format encouraged empathy, critical thinking, and deeper engagement with the subject matter, demonstrating its value not only as a research output but also as a pedagogical resource.

While photo-diaries tend to provide deep insights into individual experiences, photobooks can offer a broader overview of the research topic by collectively presenting, for example, photographs from different research participants in a visually collective manner. For this reason, photobooks are ideal for collaborative research by involving research participants in decision-making, for example, regarding the theme and the structure/layout of the photobook. Research participants can also determine how the photographs will be organised and what narratives or other additional elements will accompany them, if any.

The process of creating the photobook is an invaluable opportunity for researchers to explore how participants collectively make sense of their experiences and negotiate meanings. The process can be aided by using design software or tools available via the Internet, with or without subscription, for example, Canva®, Mixbook®, Snapfish®, and Journi®, to create a professional look.

The content of the photobooks can be reviewed for accuracy, coherence, and relevance, and the text proofread for grammatical errors at the editing stage, often AI-assisted. Printing photo-books can increase the research budget, particularly if professional printing services are involved. Options such as self-publishing platforms can be considered as well, including digital versions that are more sustainable and easier to distribute compared to physical copies.

Storyboards

Storyboards are alternative visual representations of health-related narratives, similar to a comic strip, where each frame or panel represents a key moment in the story of health or illness. As with photo-diaries and photobooks, storyboards can be used creatively to illustrate patient journeys, healthcare processes, or the impact of healthcare interventions. They provide visual clarity by breaking down complex processes into visual segments, which helps in understanding and communicating health or healthcare scenarios. This aspect is of methodological importance, particularly when narrative inquiry frameworks are incorporated, looking not only at the story content but also how the research participants tell their stories.

Storyboards can be individual, created by each research participant, or collective. The approach might be dictated by the research methodology used, for example, one-to-one interviews, creative workshops, or a combination of those. Regardless of the approach chosen, the research participants can be actively involved in designing each frame of the storyboard, focusing on key moments of their journey and transitions. To aid the process, the research participants can sketch rough drafts of each frame and integrate text or meaningful messages to provide context and make the storytelling more impactful (Figure 6.2).

More recently, photography-based storyboards have been used in quality improvements in healthcare, as illustrated in a study by Mathura et al. (2020). In this work, the authors integrated photovoice into traditional healthcare quality improvement storyboards to enhance their

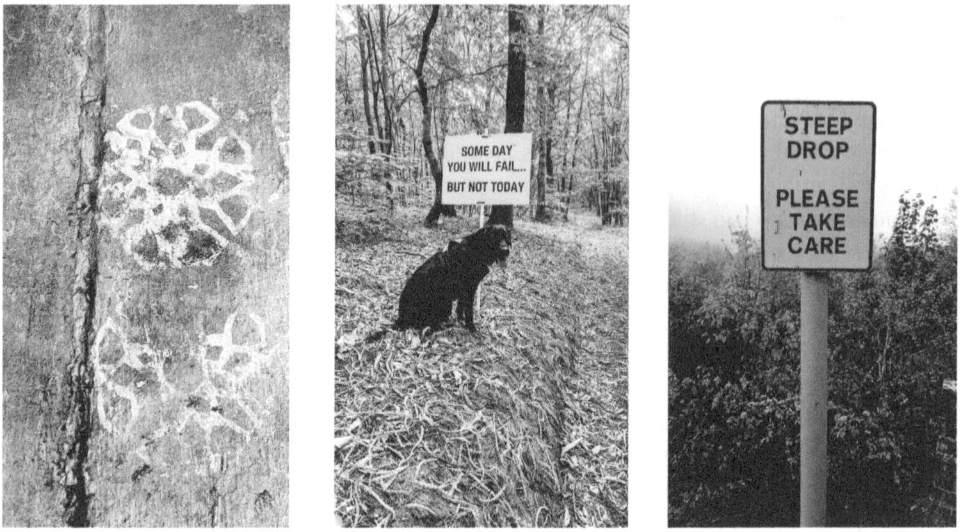
SOME DAY
YOU WILL FAIL...
BUT NOT TODAY
STEEP
DROP
PLEASE
TAKE
CARE

Past – "Snowflakes"	**Present – "Path"**	**Future – "Take care"**
I was told in whispers, as winter pressed its cruel breath against my vision, that my strength would melt – one flake at a time. And then I saw the cracks – hairline fractures, fragile architecture, splintering reflections of my days, and nights, a strange art – geometry of weakness.	I learned that failure is a season, a winter that waits beyond the bend – but not today. Today is autumn, and the path hums with hope and rustling leaves. Today, I take the path one step at a time, each step a quiet rebellion against my illness.	Fragility has a language I've been learning, warning signs nailed to a post, shouting what my body whispers. I trace the letters like cracks in ice (or is it the crystal ball?), knowing one slip could scatter me into a thousand shards. So I walk, carrying the cracks like maps, toward a horizon stitched with uncertainty.

FIGURE 6.2 Storyboard

Source: photographs and narrative by the Author

communicative power. By incorporating photographs taken by healthcare staff, the storyboards conveyed not only data and outcomes but also the emotional and contextual dimensions of care delivery. This approach helped humanise quality improvement efforts, enhanced engagement among stakeholders, and made the storyboards more accessible and impactful for diverse audiences, including patients, families, and frontline staff.

Collages

Collages can be an alternative, equally powerful and versatile tool for showcasing and disseminating photography-based research in healthcare. By combining multiple images, texts, and other visual elements into a single cohesive piece, collages can effectively communicate complex ideas and narratives (Højring & Bech-Danielsen, 2021).

Collages can attract attention and evoke emotional responses, which is crucial for conveying human aspects of healthcare experiences in a way that is inclusive and accessible. This is because collage-making does not require specialised artistic skills, which makes them an excellent medium for creatively involving participants from diverse backgrounds in the research process.

For example, family caregivers and patients can contribute their own photographs and stories, which can then be integrated into collages to reflect their unique perspectives on the research phenomena. This participatory approach not only enriches the research but also empowers participants by giving them a voice. Collages also provide an opportunity to highlight marginalised voices and experiences that might otherwise be overlooked in traditional research dissemination methods. Gorman et al. (2024) illustrate this in their study on rare diseases, where families affected by such conditions participated in a series of collage workshops. Through creative processes, participants were able to express complex emotions and experiences such as challenges of being heard, navigating treatments, and balancing care with everyday life, in ways that traditional interviews might not have captured. Collages serve as both expressive tools and analytical artefacts, offering a rich, multi-layered understanding of health and illness, as exemplified in Figures 6.3 and 6.4.

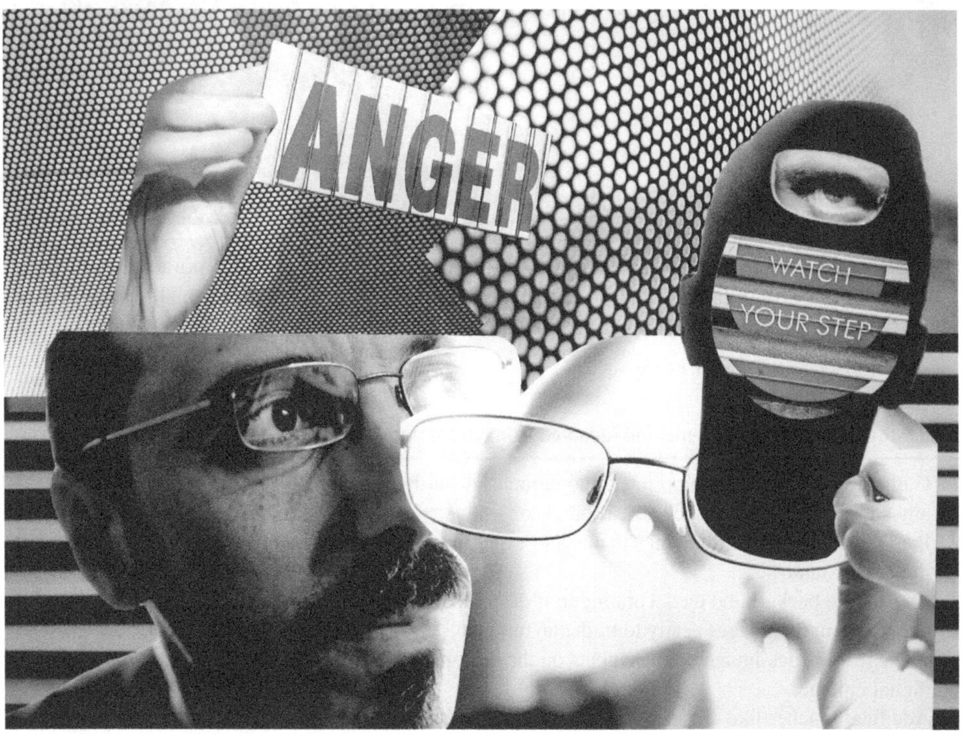

FIGURE 6.3 "Fragmentarium" – a collage of images, feelings, and thoughts surrounding living with the ocular symptoms of myasthenia gravis

Source: photographs and collage by the Author

In the context of healthcare, collages can serve as an effective knowledge translation tool that can be used in various settings, such as conferences, public art galleries, and workshops. Furthermore, creating a collage can be a fun and creative process involving several steps illustrated in Table 6.1.

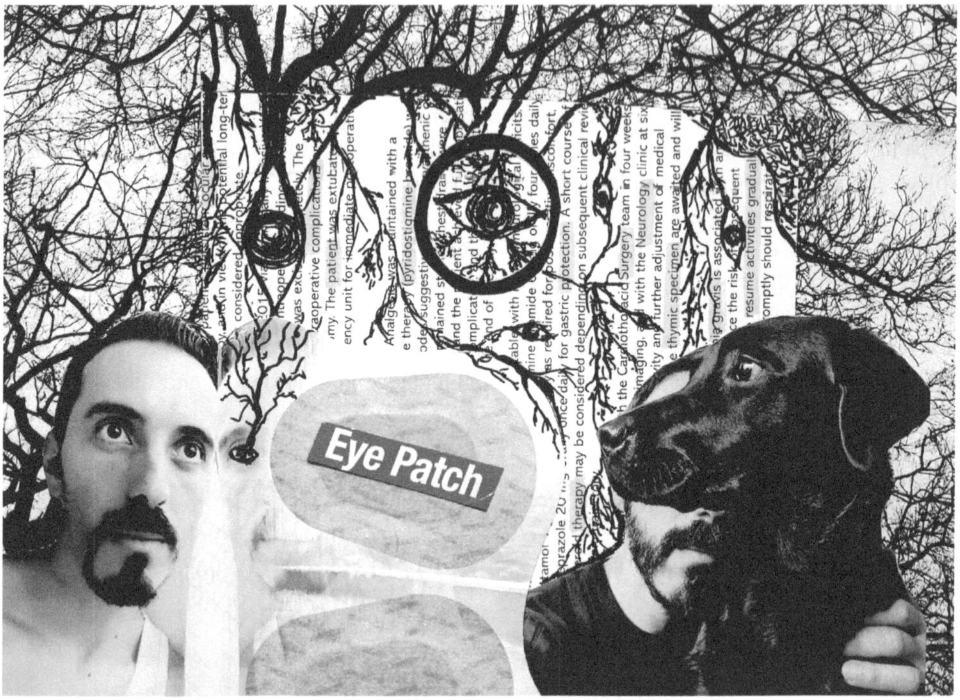

FIGURE 6.4 "Eye (I) Patch – A Patchy Past": a mixed-media collage incorporating photographs, adhesive plasters, and doodles that echo the metaphorical "neuronal" structure of the trees depicted, and a medical letter in the background

Source: photographs and collage by the Author

TABLE 6.1 Steps for collage-making (adapted from Brommer, 1994)

1. Gather materials, including printed photographs, a sturdy background e.g., cardboard, adhesives, and any additional elements such as text or stickers.
2. Plan the layout by deciding on a theme and experimenting with different arrangements of images on the background.
3. Prepare the background by decorating it, if desired, and allowing it to dry completely.
4. Cut and trim the images neatly to fit the layout plan.
5. Arrange and stick images and elements on the background using glue or tape, or digital tools for a digital collage.
6. Add final touches like text or embellishments to enhance the collage and considering sealing it with a clear varnish or mod podge for protection.
7. Review the collage for any adjustments and making necessary tweaks to ensure everything looks cohesive and balanced.
8. Display the collage by framing it and sharing it with others, depending on case, either physically or digitally.

6.2.2 *Interactive presentations*

Conference presentations

Conference oral presentations or posters are ideal opportunities for disseminating findings from photographic healthcare research. They allow for real-time interaction with the audience, facilitating discussions, questions, and feedback, which can enhance the impact and reach of the research. Additionally, presenting at conferences can lead to publication opportunities, as many conferences have associated journals or proceedings where researchers can publish their work.

Conferences are ideal opportunities to showcase photographic research by incorporating visual aids in slides designed with software such as Microsoft PowerPoint®, Prezi®, or Canva® to create visually appealing content. Furthermore, research participants can be invited to conferences as part of the audience, if they prefer to stay anonymous, or active presenters of their work, if they wish to get involved, with ethical clearance.

Feedback from conferences is key to capturing the impact of research on the target audience and improving future research, particularly for funded projects that require impact case studies. To support this, visual tools such as posters (Figure 6.5) play a vital role in communicating findings and engaging stakeholders.

Exhibitions

In-person exhibitions are another dynamic and impactful method for disseminating photography-based research. Exhibitions can provide a tangible and immersive experience, allowing viewers to interact with the photographs and, consequently, research findings. The physical presence of photographs, combined with thoughtful curation and presentation, can evoke strong emotional responses and create a deeper connection to the research topic.

Furthermore, by bringing people together in a shared space, exhibitions encourage conversations and reflections on the research topics. This interaction can lead to new insights, collaborations, and a broader understanding of the healthcare issues being presented. By displaying images alongside contextual information, such as captions or audio recordings, exhibitions can highlight the lived experiences of research participants.

Nault Connors et al. (2019) demonstrated this in their use of photovoice to engage stakeholders in planning for patient-centred outcomes research. Their project culminated in a public exhibition of participant-generated photographs and narratives, which not only facilitated meaningful dialogue among patients, caregivers, and researchers but also helped shape future research priorities by centring the voices of those with lived experience.

Similarly, in the "Amplifying the Lived Experiences of Community Health Workers (ALEC)" study (Ibe et al., 2023), community health workers in Baltimore, US, used photovoice to document their daily realities. Their photographs and stories were curated into a public exhibition titled "More Than Conquerors", displayed at the Baltimore Museum of Art. This served both as a research output and an advocacy tool, drawing attention to social determinants of health affecting communities and amplifying voices that are often underrepresented in the healthcare discourse.

In-person exhibitions can attract a wide range of audiences, from local community members to international attendees, depending on the venue and promotion. This broad reach helps to disseminate research findings to a diverse audience, increasing awareness and understanding

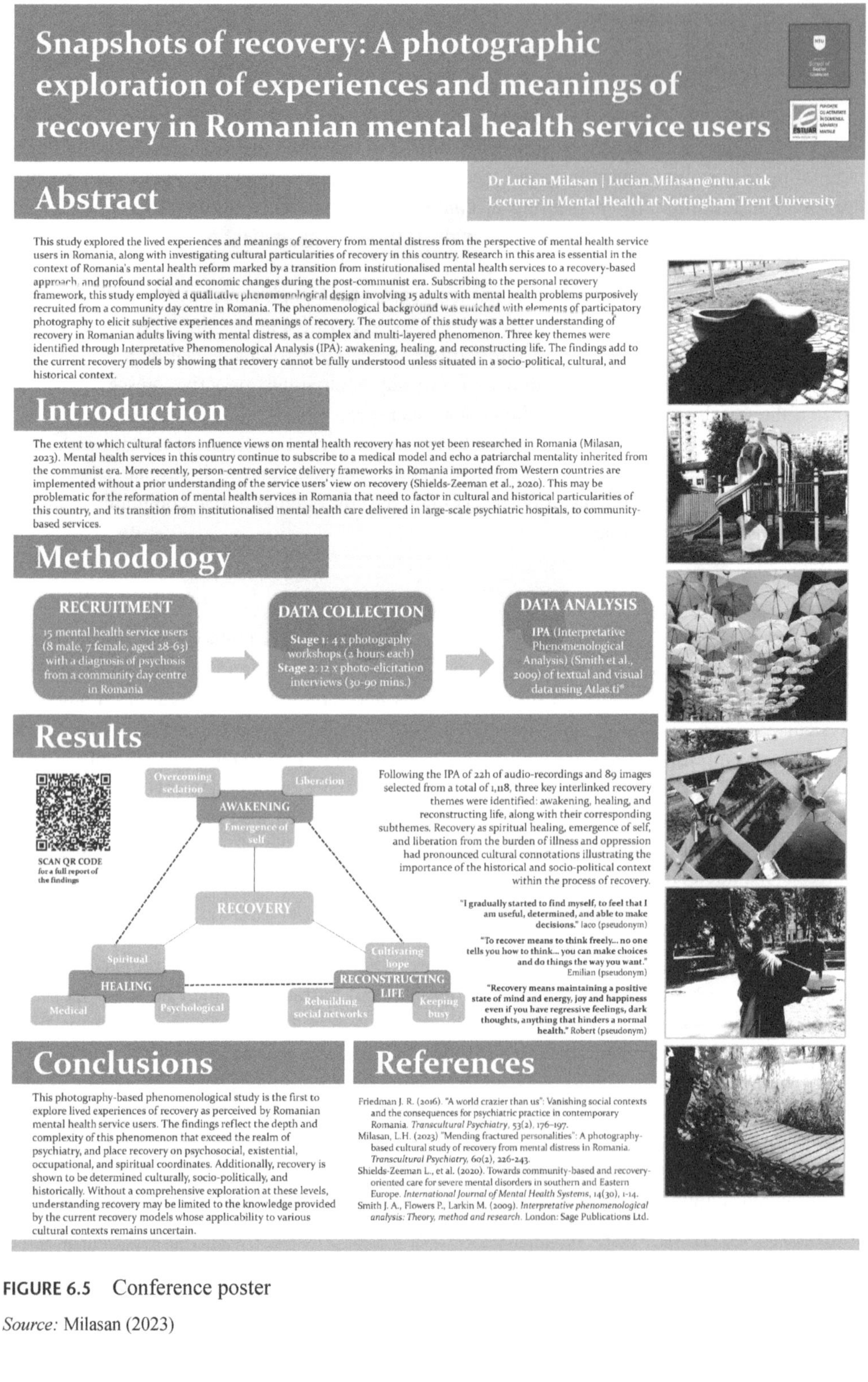

FIGURE 6.5 Conference poster

Source: Milasan (2023)

of important healthcare topics. Additionally, exhibitions can be held in various settings, such as hospitals, universities, galleries, and public spaces, making the research accessible to different communities.

Complementing these physical spaces, online photo exhibitions have emerged as effective and accessible platforms for showcasing photography-based research. Online exhibitions remove geographical barriers to participation, resulting in expanding the reach of the research to a wider and potentially more diverse audience. Furthermore, online exhibitions can incorporate interactive elements that enhance viewer engagement. Features such as clickable images, embedded videos, and virtual tours allow viewers to explore the research in a more dynamic and immersive manner. These interactive formats can make complex healthcare topics more understandable and engaging, which is conducive to a deeper connection to the research.

A compelling example is the "Co-PACT Photovoice" online exhibition (University of Oxford, 2023) involving over 60 participants with lived experience of detention under the Mental Health Act. A curated selection of these images was presented in an online photovoice gallery (link provided with the reference), offering powerful visual narratives that highlight systemic inequalities and personal experiences within mental health care. The digital format allowed for wide accessibility and served as a platform for advocacy, reflection, and policy engagement.

Hosting an online exhibition is often more cost-effective and sustainable compared to traditional in-person exhibitions with platforms such as Flickr®, Google Sites®, and Artsteps® offering free or low-cost options for creating and sharing digital exhibitions. As there are no expenses related to venue rental, transportation, or physical setup, this option is attractive for researchers with limited budgets. Additionally, online exhibitions have a lower environmental impact, as they do not require physical materials or travel.

Furthermore, online exhibitions can remain accessible for extended periods, allowing viewers to revisit the content at their convenience. This continuous access ensures research remains available to new audiences over time, while researchers can update and expand the exhibition content as new findings emerge, keeping the information current and relevant.

Virtual platforms for online exhibitions can facilitate collaboration and networking among researchers, people with lived experience of accessing health services, healthcare professionals, and other stakeholders. Features such as discussion forums, often with moderation, live chats, and webinars, can be integrated into online exhibitions, providing opportunities for real-time interaction and knowledge exchange. As a result, this collaborative environment can lead to new partnerships and advancements in healthcare research.

Virtual/Augmented Reality

Virtual Reality (VR) and Augmented Reality (AR) are transformative technologies that offer innovative and immersive ways to engage audiences, enhance understanding, and facilitate interaction with research content. In immersive VR environments, users can explore photographic research in a three-dimensional space and interact with images and narratives in a life-like setting (Setyawan et al., 2023). Augmented Reality, on the other hand, overlays digital elements onto the real world, enhancing the viewer's experience by adding contextual information and interactive features (Lee et al., 2024).

By allowing viewers to interact with photographic data, these technologies can make abstract concepts more relatable and easier to grasp. For example, viewers can zoom in on images, access detailed descriptions, and view related multimedia content, all within the immersive environment.

As with online exhibitions hosted by a variety of websites and platforms, VR and AR platforms can facilitate remote access to exhibitions, making them accessible to a global audience. Additionally, these technologies support real-time collaboration and interaction. Features such as virtual meetings, live chats, and collaborative workspaces allow stakeholders to discuss and analyse research findings together within an interactive research environment.

The use of VR and AR in healthcare research and practice is rapidly expanding. These technologies are being used for medical training, patient education, pain management, and rehabilitation (Yeung et al., 2021). In the context of photographic research, VR and AR can create virtual galleries, interactive case studies, and immersive storytelling experiences that showcase key research findings and insights, with potential impact on enhancing healthcare practices.

6.2.3 Digital repositories

Digital repositories are essential tools for storing, organising, and disseminating photography-based research. These digital platforms offer numerous advantages, including easy access, efficient management, and enhanced collaboration. Digital repositories provide a centralised location for storing large collections of digital photographs and related data, otherwise difficult to manage. Photographs can be organised with metadata, that is, information such as camera settings, date and time the photo was taken, location (GPS coordinates), and copyright information, alongside tags and descriptions, all within ethical parameters. This can facilitate efficient searching and sorting of photographs, making it easier for researchers to locate specific images or datasets.

Shared digital repositories can also facilitate effective collaboration among researchers and institutions. By providing secure access to shared resources, these platforms allow multiple users to contribute, annotate, and analyse photographs collectively, regardless of their location. Furthermore, virtual repositories can integrate with various analytical tools and software, enhancing the ability to collaboratively analyse and interpret photographic data.

Virtual repositories ensure long-term preservation of photographic data. By storing images in secure, cloud-based systems, these platforms protect against data loss due to hardware failures or other physical risks to which researchers are often exposed. This is because repositories often include backup and recovery features, ensuring that data remains safe and accessible over time.

Many virtual repositories offer open access options, allowing researchers to share their photographic data with a global audience. Open access repositories promote transparency and reproducibility in research, enabling other scientists to validate findings and build upon existing work, which is a key aspect in contemporary research. A prime example is the National Library of Medicine's (2026) Historical Photographs Collection (link provided in the reference), which houses thousands of digitised images documenting the history of medicine, public health, and healthcare practices. This repository demonstrates how photographs can be preserved, enriched with metadata, and made accessible to researchers, educators, and the public.

6.2.4 Social media

Social media has become an indispensable tool for showcasing and disseminating photography-based research in healthcare (Kia-Keating et al., 2017). Photography-based research is particularly well-suited for social media and blogs due to the visual nature of these platforms. Social media platforms offer a range of advantages, including broad reach, interactive engagement, and real-time communication. For example, Instagram, Facebook, X, and LinkedIn have almost 7 billion users combined, allowing researchers to break geographical barriers of more conventional showcase events like in-person exhibitions. This broad reach ensures that important healthcare topics gain visibility and awareness across different communities, including hard-to-reach populations (Wright et al., 2024).

Social media facilitates interactive engagement with viewers through features such as comments, likes, shares, and direct messaging, which enables real-time interaction and feedback. Researchers can use these tools to engage with their audience, answer questions, and promote discussions about their findings. This interactive approach not only supports understanding but also builds a sense of community around research. By combining photographs with captions, infographics, and videos, researchers can create engaging content that resonates with viewers and makes their research more impactful (Bardus et al., 2020).

Social media allows researchers to share new developments, preliminary results, and ongoing projects as they happen. Additionally, social media algorithms and the use of hashtags can amplify the reach of posts, ensuring that content is seen by larger audiences and easily tracked through built-in analytics and dedicated monitoring tools. Furthermore, social media provides an effective platform for networking with other professionals nationally and internationally, enabling connections that can advance research and career development.

Conclusion

Effective reporting and dissemination can transform photography-based research from a static record into a dynamic tool for knowledge exchange, policy influence, and meaningful change in healthcare practice. However, reporting and disseminating findings from photography-based research requires more than simply presenting images alongside text. A clear rationale for using photographic techniques strengthens the credibility of the study, while detailed documentation of processes ensures reproducibility and trustworthiness. Integrating visual and textual data in a coherent narrative is essential for conveying depth and authenticity. Beyond traditional academic outputs, innovative dissemination strategies such as photobooks, storyboards, collages, exhibitions, and digital platforms, offer opportunities to amplify participant voices and extend the reach of research.

Knowledge check

1. Why is it important to articulate a clear rationale for using photographic techniques in healthcare research?
2. What are some common pitfalls when presenting photographic findings, and how can they be avoided?
3. What are some creative and innovative methods for disseminating photography-based research findings, and how might they enhance audience engagement?
4. In what ways can the integration of visual and textual elements in dissemination strategies improve (or hinder) the accessibility and emotional resonance of research findings?

References

Achiam, M., Vitting-Seerup, S., Hurley, M., Grimaud, C. M., Chanay, R., Erić, D. L., Laursen, S., Dunets, V., & Russo, P. (2025). Practical rationales for art-science in science communication. *International Journal of Science Education, Part B*, 1–14. https://doi.org/10.1080/21548455.2025.2523572

Alves, K. Y. A., Rodrigues, C. C. F. M., Salvador, P. T. C. O., & Fernandes, S. D. M. (2021). Use of photography in qualitative research in the health area: Scoping review. *Ciência & Saúde Coletiva, 26*(2), 521–529. https://doi.org/10.1590/1413-81232021262.41052020

Bardus, M., El Rassi, R., Chahrour, M., Akl, E. W., Raslan, A. S., Meho, L. I., & Akl, E. A. (2020). The use of social media to increase the impact of health research: Systematic review. *Journal of Medical Internet Research, 22*(7), e15607. https://doi.org/10.2196/15607

Bolaki, S. (2016). Capturing the worlds of multiple sclerosis: Hannah Laycock's photography. *Medical Humanities, 43*(1), 47–54. https://doi.org/10.1136/medhum-2016-011073

Brommer, G. F. (1994). *Collage techniques: A guide for artists and illustrators.* Watson-Guptill Publications.

Brooks, S. P., Zimmermann, G. L., Lang, M., Scott, S. D., Thomson, D., Wilkes, G., & Hartling, L. (2022). A framework to guide storytelling as a knowledge translation intervention for health-promoting behaviour change. *Implementation Science Communications, 3*(35), 1–13. https://doi.org/10.1186/s43058-022-00282-6

Cleland, J., & MacLeod, A. (2021). The visual vernacular: Embracing photographs in research. *Perspectives in Medical Education, 10*(1), 230–237. https://doi.org/10.1007/s40037-021-00672-x

Davda, M., & Pasquali, P. (2020). Standardization in photographic documentation. In P. Pasquali (Ed.), *Photography in clinical medicine* (pp. 211–230). Springer. https://doi.org/10.1007/978-3-030-24544-3_14

Dodd, S., Carter, G., Christie, A., & Mitchell, G. (2022). Exploring nurse and nursing student experience of using an artist-produced photobook to learn about dementia. *BMC Nursing, 21*(1), 1–12. https://doi.org/10.1186/s12912-022-00991-2

Gorman, R., Farsides, B., & Bonner, M. (2024). Crafting representations of rare disease: Collage as qualitative inquiry. *Arts & Health, 16*(3), 285–302. https://doi.org/10.1080/17533015.2023.2254328

Gurrieri, L., & Drenten, J. (2019). Visual storytelling and vulnerable health care consumers: Normalising practices and social support through Instagram. *Journal of Services Marketing, 33*(6), 696–706. https://doi.org/10.1108/JSM-09-2018-0262

Harris, P., Ellem, K., Gallagher, H., Burgess, A., Abson, L., & Sunderland, N. (2022). Building capacity to engage in co-produced research: Reflections from a digital storytelling project. *Disability & Society, 39*(5), 1256–275. https://doi.org/10.1080/09687599.2022.2138267

Holm, G. (2014). Photography as a research method. In P. Leavy (Ed.), *The Oxford handbook of qualitative research* (pp. 380–402). Oxford University Press. https://doi.org/10.1093/oxfordhb/9780199811755.013.031

Højring, L. H., & Bech-Danielsen, C. (2021). Homelessness and homeliness: Collage technique as a research method. In V. Buchli (Ed.), *Architectural anthropology: Exploring lived space* (pp. 76–89). Routledge.

Ibe, C., Hines, A., Carrero, N. D., Fuller, S., Trainor, A., Scott, T., Hickman, D., & Cooper, L. A. (2023). Voices, images, and experiences of community health workers: Advancing antiracist policy and practice. *Health Affairs, 42*(10), 1392–1401. https://doi.org/10.1377/hlthaff.2023.00584

Kia-Keating, M., Santacrose, D., & Liu, S. (2017). Photography and social media use in community-based participatory research with youth: Ethical considerations. *American Journal of Community Psychology, 60*(3–4), 375–384. https://doi.org/10.1002/ajcp.12189

Kuo, M. C., Chen, C. M., Wu, F. G., Chen, C. H., Yin, Z. X., & Wang, C. Y. (2022). Use of photo diary and focus group to explore needs for digital disease management program among community older adults with chronic disease. *Health & Social Care in the Community, 30*(3), 926–936. https://doi.org/10.1111/hsc.13241

Langmann, S., & Pick, D. (2018). Ethical considerations in photography as a research method. In *Photography as a social research method* (pp. 35–52). Springer. https://doi.org/10.1007/978-981-10-7279-6_3

Lee, C.-I., Pan, Y.-H., & Chen, B. (2024). Participatory exhibition-viewing using augmented reality and analysis of visitor behavior. *Applied Sciences, 14*(9), 1–14. https://doi.org/10.3390/app14093579

Mathura, P., Li, M., McMurtry, N., & Kassam, N. (2020). Enhancing the healthcare quality improvement storyboard using photovoice. *BMJ Open Quality, 9*(4), e001104. https://doi.org/10.1136/bmjoq-2020-001104

Milasan, L. H. (2023). *Snapshots of recovery: A photographic exploration of experiences and meanings of recovery in Romanian mental health service users* (conference poster). 6–7 September 2023.

National Library of Medicine. (2026). *Historical photographs collection.* https://www.nlm.nih.gov/hmd/collections/photos.html

Nault Connors, J. D., Conley, M. J., & Lorenz, L. S. (2019). Use of Photovoice to engage stakeholders in planning for patient-centered outcomes research. *Research Involvement and Engagement, 5*(1), 1–10. https://doi.org/10.1186/s40900-019-0166-y

Newransky, C., Adames-Torres, J., Lloyd, S., Benash, S. B., & Rozario, P. (2024). Café Photovoice: A participatory approach to program evaluation in community mental health in the United States. In M. Florence, W. Vanderplasschen, M. Yu, J. D. Maeyer, & S. Savahl (Eds.), *Handbook of addiction, recovery and quality of life* (pp. 243–255). Springer. https://doi.org/10.1007/978-3-031-65873-0_16
NHS (University Hospitals of Morecambe Bay). (2021). *Lucy's photobook brings a ray of sunshine to hospital patients*. https://www.uhmb.nhs.uk/news-and-events/latest-news/lucys-photobook-brings-ray-sunshine-hospital-patients
Ntsobi, M. P., Costa, A. P., Kasperiuniene, J., Brandão, C., & Ribeiro, J. (2024). Digital tools and techniques in qualitative research: Digital skills and research optimisation. In J. Ribeiro, C. Brandão, M. Ntsobi, J. Kasperiuniene, & A. P. Costa (Eds.), *Computer supported qualitative research* (pp. 1–25). Springer.
Olmos-Vega, F. M., Stalmeijer, R. E., Varpio, L., & Kahlke, R. (2023). A practical guide to reflexivity in qualitative research. *Medical Teacher, 45*(3), 241–251. https://doi.org/10.1080/0142159X.2022.2057287
Parr, M., & Badger, G. (2004). *The photobook: A history* (Vol. 1). Phaidon.
Pasquali, P. (2020). *Photography in clinical medicine*. Springer.
Richard, V. M., & Lahman, M. K. E. (2015). Photo-elicitation: Reflexivity on method, analysis, and graphic portraits. *International Journal of Research & Method in Education, 38*(1), 3–22. https://doi.org/10.1080/1743727X.2013.843073
Schrader, S. M., Deering, E. N., Zahl, D. A., & Wallace, M. (2011). Visually storying living with HIV: Bridging stressors and supports in accessing care. *Health Education Research, 26*(4), 638–652. https://doi.org/10.1093/her/cyr023
Setyawan, R. S., Hidayat, M. M., Febrianti, L., & Firmansyah, M. A. (2023). Implementation of virtual reality for photography exhibitions. *Journal of Electrical Engineering and Computer Sciences, 8*(1), 1–7. https://doi.org/10.54732/jeecs.v8i1.6
Sitvast, J. E., & Springer, W. (2020). The use of photography in perceiving a sense in life: A phenomenological and existential approach in mental health care. *Nursing Philosophy, 21*(2), e12287. https://doi.org/10.1111/nup.12287
Trombeta, G., & Cox, S. M. (2022). The Textual-Visual Thematic Analysis: A framework to analyze the conjunction and interaction of visual and textual data. *The Qualitative Report, 27*(6), 1557–1574. https://doi.org/10.46743/2160-3715/2022.5456
University of Oxford. (2023). *Photovoice Exhibition – Experiences of people detained under the Mental Health Act*. https://www.psych.ox.ac.uk/research/chimes/co-pact/photovoice-exhibition
Utomo, A., Grant, C., & Grundy, J. (2025). Team photo-diaries as a method for collaborative reflection in a community health census in Cambodia. *Global Health Action, 18*(1), 1234567. https://doi.org/10.1111/1745-5871.70020
Volpe, C. R. (2019). Digital diaries: New uses of PhotoVoice in participatory research with young people. *Children's Geographies, 17*(3), 361–370. https://doi.org/10.1080/14733285.2018.1543852
Wright, A. L., Willett, Y. J., Ferron, E. M., Kumarasamy, V., Lem, S. M., & Ahmed, O. (2024). Using social media to recruit participants in health care research: Case study. *Journal of Medical Internet Research, 26*(1), e51751. https://doi.org/10.2196/51751
Yeung, A. W. K., Tosevska, A., Klager, E., Eibensteiner, F., Laxar, D., Stoyanov, J., Glisic, M., Zeiner, S., Kulnik, S. T., Crutzen, R., Kimberger, O., Kletecka-Pulker, M., Atanasov, A. G., & Willschke, H. (2021). Virtual and augmented reality applications in medicine: Analysis of the scientific literature. *Journal of Medical Internet Research, 23*(2), e25499. https://doi.org/10.2196/25499
Young, R., Dongilli, D., Souder, A., & Peek-Asa, C. (2024). Stories for us, or for others: Digital storytelling with a harm reduction organization as culture-centered health communication. *Health Communication, 40*(8), 1465–1478. https://doi.org/10.1080/10410236.2024.2405767

Further reading

Williamson, I. R., Quincey, K., Lond, B. J., & Papaloukas, P. (2021). Unanticipated voices? Reflections from our ongoing 'adventures' with participant-authored photography, interviewing and interpretative phenomenology. *Methods in Psychology, 5*(1), 100062. https://doi.org/10.1016/j.metip.2021.100062

7

ETHICS IN HEALTH RESEARCH USING PHOTOGRAPHIC TECHNIQUES

7.1 Ethical foundations of photography-based healthcare research

Healthcare research – whether or not it involves photographic methods – is fundamentally guided by ethical principles designed to safeguard the rights, dignity, and well-being of participants. This chapter is structured around the four core principles of biomedical ethics as outlined by Beauchamp and Childress (1989): autonomy, non-maleficence, beneficence, and justice, and how they may link to photographic research. In a nutshell, *autonomy* is reflected in the participant's control over how their image is captured, used, and shared. *Non-maleficence* involves minimising potential harm that may arise from visual exposure, misrepresentation, or unintended dissemination. *Beneficence* is evident in the therapeutic and expressive potential of photography, particularly in participatory research where individuals can visually articulate their health experiences. Finally, *justice* requires equitable representation and fair treatment of research participants in photography-based research. Together, these principles provide a valuable and critical ethical framework for designing and conducting photography-based research in healthcare settings.

7.1.1 Autonomy

Autonomy is a fundamental principle in healthcare research ethics, requiring that participants are respected as self-determining agents capable of making informed decisions about their involvement in research. In the context of photography-based research, this principle takes on particular significance, as participants are not simply subjects but active contributors to visual narratives that may reflect intimate aspects of their health and identity.

Respect for autonomy entails more than informed consent; it involves promoting genuine agency. This includes ensuring that participants understand the purpose of the research, the role of photographic methods, their benefits and challenges, how images will be used, and who the potential audiences may be. Informed consent must be an ongoing, dialogic process, not a one-time transaction. Participants should retain the right to opt out or withdraw at any stage,

DOI: 10.4324/9781003537540-8

and their preferences regarding image use and representation must be prioritised throughout the research lifecycle.

Particular attention must be given to individuals who may have limited capacity for autonomous decision-making, such as children, those with cognitive impairments, mental health conditions, or learning disabilities. In such cases, researchers must take additional steps to ensure that participation is both ethical and empowering, rather than inadvertently reinforcing vulnerability (Hamilton et al., 2017). Visual consent forms using images, icons, or simplified diagrams can support understanding and engagement, especially for children or individuals with cognitive or communication challenges, by making the consent process more accessible and meaningful (Berti Suman, 2024).

Autonomy also extends to decisions about representation. Participants should have control over how they and their experiences are portrayed in visual outputs. This includes the right to review and approve photographs prior to dissemination. Such practices not only uphold ethical standards but also encourage trust and collaboration between researchers and participants (Langmann & Pick, 2017).

As Ponic and Jategaonkar (2012) argue, autonomy is centrally concerned with self-determination and choice, but must be understood within the broader socio-economic, cultural, and political contexts in which participants live. A relational perspective on autonomy supported by Bergum and Dossetor (2005) highlights the influence of interpersonal dynamics and societal structures on decision-making. Sherwin (1998) cautions that treating autonomy as an isolated, individual act risks obscuring the power relations and structural inequalities that shape participants' choices. In photography-based healthcare research, acknowledging these contextual factors is essential to ensuring that autonomy is not only respected in theory but also enacted in practice.

Researchers can support autonomy in practice by incorporating co-design approaches, where participants help shape the research process, and by facilitating image review sessions that allow individuals to reflect on, approve, or revise how their visual narratives are represented and disseminated. This approach is exemplified in Barry et al.'s (2021) photovoice project involving service users and family members to co-produce and co-facilitate a mental health education intervention. In this study, participants were actively involved in co-producing and curating a public exhibition, thereby retaining decision-making power from the project's inception to its conclusion, and reinforcing autonomy through collaborative practice.

7.1.2 Non-maleficence

Non-maleficence – the ethical obligation to avoid causing harm – is another key principle in healthcare practice and research. Harm can manifest in various forms, including physical injury, emotional distress, social repercussions such as discrimination or the unintended disclosure of sensitive information, and legal consequences such as breaches of legislation concerning privacy and other human rights. Importantly, harm may affect not only individual participants but also broader groups or communities. For instance, findings from photographic research that inadvertently stereotype a community can reinforce stigma and contribute to ongoing social marginalisation (Ng et al., 2023).

In photography-based research, the potential for harm extends to both participants and researchers. While photography may appear to be an innocuous method for documenting lived experiences, it can evoke powerful emotional responses. Photographs often intensify the emotional content of participants' narratives, surfacing subconscious memories and triggering distress, particularly when revisiting traumatic health experiences (Saita & Tramontano, 2018).

This emotional depth, while valuable for insight, increases the risk of psychological harm for participants and, in some cases, for researchers who engage closely with sensitive material. This is evidenced in Moncur's (2013) qualitative survey on the emotional well-being of researchers, where a participant reflected on the emotional toll of working with death-related materials: "It was very upsetting for me . . . looking at the photos and hearing the stories was terrible". In other situations, researchers may experience vicarious trauma or compassion fatigue due to their personal connection to the topic (Fahie, 2014). Moncur (2013) recommends proactive strategies to support researchers' well-being, including reflective supervision, peer support, and institutional recognition of emotional labour within research practice. This support is essential particularly when self-harm (Edmondson et al., 2018), suicide (Creighton et al., 2018a), and other sensitive topics are explored through photography.

Researchers must also consider the harm potentially caused by legal and ethical implications of encouraging participants to photograph others, especially in public or clinical settings. Without clear guidance and compliance with relevant legislation such as data protection laws in the jurisdiction where the research is conducted, participants may inadvertently violate others' privacy rights, potentially exposing themselves and the research team to legal repercussions.

7.1.3 Beneficence

At the other end of the ethical spectrum, beneficence is focused on maximising the benefits of research and promoting participant well-being. Photography is a creative and reflective practice widely recognised for its therapeutic potential within and beyond research contexts, as discussed in Chapter 1. Participants often report enhanced emotional expression, increased self-awareness, and even improved mental health as indirect outcomes of engaging with photography-based methods. These benefits are further illustrated in a study by Smith et al. (2024), which explored the use of photovoice in the context of recovery from substance use. In addition to therapeutic gains, the study highlights outcomes such as stigma reduction, advocacy, collaborative learning, and skill development. Such benefits may emerge unintentionally yet meaningfully through the processes of storytelling, visual expression, and collective dialogue.

In photovoice and photo-elicitation studies, participants frequently develop new photographic skills through training and creative workshops, as revealed in a review of photovoice in public health (Catalani & Minkler, 2010). In participatory and co-produced research, this may extend to the acquisition of research-related competencies, such as interviewing, data analysis, or public speaking – skills that can lead to an increased sense of agency and confidence (Smith et al., 2022). Furthermore, photography-based research often facilitates individual and collective learning about the research topic, such as health experiences, social and health inequities, or available community resources (Milasan, 2023).

The process of knowledge co-creation that is often at the core of photographic research can lead to personal empowerment, particularly when participants are given platforms to share their stories and promote change (Budig et al., 2018). When visual narratives are shared with wider audiences through exhibitions, community forums, or policy briefings, they can catalyse tangible outcomes, such as improved health services, increased awareness, or even policy reform. This is evident in Kramer et al.'s (2010) study, where photovoice was used within a community health initiative to engage community members in identifying local health concerns and influencing environmental and policy changes. The project not only amplified community voices but also contributed to concrete improvements in neighbourhood infrastructure and health-promoting environments, demonstrating the potential of photovoice to influence decision-makers and create opportunities for change in the health system.

7.1.4 Justice

The ethical principle of justice in research concerns the fair and equitable treatment of participants and the just distribution of research benefits. This begins with inclusive and thoughtful recruitment practices to ensure diverse voices and perspectives are represented, particularly those historically marginalised or underrepresented (Breny & McMorrow, 2021). Research often involves hard-to-reach populations or individuals experiencing a range of vulnerabilities, from socio-economic disadvantages to racial inequities and social exclusion. Upholding the principle of justice requires that photographic research actively avoids reinforcing these disparities or perpetuating stereotypes and power imbalances. Therefore, researchers must be especially cautious not to exploit marginalised groups or reproduce narratives that contribute to a sense of injustice among participants.

Photography can contribute meaningfully to this principle by functioning as a participatory research tool that amplifies the voices of those often silenced and promotes social justice through visual storytelling (Sanon et al., 2014). This is possible due to the democratisation of the photographic act, which has made image-making more accessible and inclusive. As Sankey (2014) argues, the shift from photography as an elite, highly technical practice to a widely available and expressive medium has enabled individuals from diverse backgrounds to document their realities and challenge dominant narratives. In health research, this democratisation allows participants to become co-creators of knowledge, using photography not only to reflect their lived experiences of health and illness but also to assert their identities and advocate for change on their own terms.

By grounding photographic healthcare research in these ethical foundations, researchers can uphold participant dignity, and produce meaningful, socially responsible work. This alignment strengthens the credibility and impact of research and helps the researcher address and reflect upon more practical ethical considerations. Some of these are discussed in the next section along with strategies for mitigating ethical issues in photography-based research.

7.2 Key ethical considerations in photography-based health research

Ethical considerations in photography have been a subject of concern even before photography became an established methodological tool in research. Susan Sontag (1977) highlighted the profound ethical challenges inherent in photographing and viewing images of suffering – an issue particularly relevant in the context of health and illness. Sontag argued that photography can lead to a detached, almost voyeuristic relationship with the pain and distress of others, raising concerns about potential exploitation of research participants. Such representations risk being intrusive and may portray individuals in ways that misrepresent their lived experiences. In her critical examination of photography's moral dimensions, Sontag challenged the notion of objectivity in photographic practice, asserting that the inherent subjectivity of image-making necessitates a re-evaluation of ethical responsibilities in both the production and interpretation of visual material.

Building on Sontag's foundational insights and more recent scholarship (Creighton et al., 2018b; Groot et al., 2021; Ng et al., 2023; Teti, 2019), this section critically explores the ethical complexities and dilemmas that arise in photography-based research. Key concerns include informed consent, confidentiality and privacy, anonymisation and pseudonymisation, (mis)representation, power dynamics, and issues of ownership and copyright. The discussion also considers the psychological and emotional impact of engaging with photographic methodologies on both participants and researchers. This section includes practical strategies for anticipating and mitigating ethical challenges with the aim of creating opportunities for more reflexive, respectful, and ethically sound research practices.

7.2.1 Informed consent

Informed consent is a fundamental ethical principle and a pillar of accountability in both healthcare practice and research. It is closely linked to the principle of autonomy discussed in the previous section. Informed consent ensures that individuals are fully aware of, and voluntarily agree to, their participation in a study, including how their data will be handled. In photography-based health research, where visual data can reveal deeply personal and identifiable information, the consent process must be especially robust, transparent, and ongoing.

Unlike traditional research methods, securing consent in visual methodologies is not a one-time administrative task confined to signing a consent form (see example in Table 7.1). It requires a continuous, dialogic process that ensures participants understand the purpose of the research, the potential risks and benefits, and the specific ways in which their photographs may be used. As a result, consent must be (re)negotiated throughout the research process before, during, and after fieldwork (Klykken, 2021). This includes decisions about whether images will be shared in academic publications, exhibitions, community presentations, or online platforms. To address this, researchers should adopt a flexible consent model that allows participants to revisit and revise their choices at different stages of the project, ensuring that consent remains informed, voluntary, and contextually appropriate throughout the research lifecycle. Wiertz and Boldt (2022) reviewed and evaluated a range of consent models in healthcare environments, including tiered or multi-layered consent, which gives participants the option to define the scope and specificity of their consent across different phases of the study. Researchers should also establish clear protocols for handling withdrawal of consent after images have been disseminated, including outlining the limitations of retraction in digital and public domains and offering participants options for partial withdrawal or anonymisation where full removal is not feasible (Florea, 2023).

As part of the consent process, participants should be clearly informed of the potential risks associated with public dissemination of their images, including the possibility that photographs may be copied, misused, or taken out of context. These concerns are especially pronounced in digital contexts, where image sharing is rapid, widespread, and often irreversible, underscoring the need for heightened vigilance and transparency in how consent is obtained and maintained (Roguljić et al., 2025).

In addition to these practical concerns, legal considerations further complicate the consent process. Under data protection regulations such as the GDPR, identifiable photographs are classified as personal data and require explicit consent for their use. This is particularly relevant in healthcare settings, where images may capture sensitive health-related information. In such contexts, consent must be specific, informed, freely given, and clearly documented, with

TABLE 7.1 Example of consent form

Consent Form

Project Title: Visual Narratives of Patient Experiences in Chronic Illness Management

Thank you for your interest in participating in this research project, which aims to explore patient experiences in managing chronic illnesses using photography as a research method. The findings will contribute to improving patient-centred care and support systems.

Before consenting to participate, please read the participant information sheet and initial each box below if you agree. If you have any questions, please speak to [insert contact details here].

Please initial each statement:

- I confirm that I have read the participant information sheet and understand the research aim and my role.
- I have had the opportunity to ask questions about my participation and have received satisfactory answers.
- I understand that my participation will be audio-recorded and transcribed using a pseudonym (made-up name) of my choice to protect my identity.
- I understand that audio-recordings will be kept until the research project is examined and then disposed of securely.
- I understand that my participation is voluntary.
- I understand that I can withdraw at any time without giving a reason and without affecting my legal rights.
- I understand that once my contributions are anonymised and incorporated into themes, it may not be possible to withdraw my data after three months after the interview, but every attempt will be made by the research team to extract it.
- I understand that I can take pictures of recognisable people only with their written consent using the provided consent form, and that recognisable faces will be anonymised by the researcher.
- I consent to my contributions being used anonymously in publications, reports, presentations, conferences, training events, discussions with policymakers, books, and for educational purposes.
- I understand the risk of my photographs being copied and shared beyond the researcher's control, once publicised.
- I understand that my information will remain confidential and anonymous unless there is a risk of harm, in which case the researcher may need to share it with their supervisor or relevant authorities.
- I consent to the research keeping anonymised transcriptions of my contributions for five years after the study is completed.
- I confirm I am 18 years old or older.
- I consent to take part in the above study.

(N.B. two copies i.e., one for the participant and one for the researcher should be signed)

Participant's Name: ________________ **Signature:** ________________ **Date:** ______
Researcher's Name: ________________ **Signature:** ________________ **Date:** ______

participants fully understanding how their images will be used, the scope of dissemination, and their right to withdraw consent at any point.

Exceptions may apply in public spaces where individuals are incidental to the image. However, these vary by jurisdiction from country to country and must be approached with caution. In private spaces, including hospitals, clinics, and care homes, permission from institutional management or property owners is also required. Participants should be made aware of these legal boundaries and potential consequences of non-compliance, including breaches of confidentiality, reputational harm, and legal liability. Researchers must therefore ensure consent procedures are not only ethically sound but also legally compliant, particularly when working in sensitive or regulated environments, which is often the case with healthcare settings.

Photography-based research often involves vulnerable populations, including children, individuals with mental health conditions, and older adults. In such cases, additional safeguards are necessary. For minors, informed consent must be obtained from a parent or legal guardian, and assent should be sought from the child in an age-appropriate manner. For example, in a health promotion study on photovoice with primary school children, Abma et al. (2022) emphasised the importance of a carefully structured consent process that respects both legal rights and the evolving capacities of children. They highlighted that informed consent in such contexts must go beyond formal documentation to include ongoing dialogue with both children and their guardians. The researchers found that while children were eager to participate and share their photo-stories, it was essential to ensure they fully understood the implications of their involvement, including how their images and narratives might be used. This requires clear, age-appropriate explanations and repeated opportunities for children to ask questions or withdraw.

Similarly, for individuals with limited mental capacity, researchers must assess the need for guardian consent and ensure that ethical protections are in place, including adherence to institutional safeguarding policies and background checks where appropriate. This is often the case with photography-based research in dementia, where cognitive fluctuations may affect participants' ability to fully comprehend the implications of their involvement. As Wiersma (2011) notes, such research requires a sensitive and flexible consent process prioritising participants' dignity, autonomy, and evolving capacity to engage meaningfully throughout the study.

To address these complexities, many researchers adopt a multi-stage consent process. This typically includes initial written consent outlining the study's aims and risks, consent forms for individuals who may appear in participants' photographs, and final consent regarding the release and use of creative materials. Written consent is often revisited and verbally reaffirmed at key stages of research, such as before or after interviews, during image selection, and prior to dissemination. This iterative approach allows participants to reflect on their involvement and make informed decisions as the project evolves (Xu et al., 2020).

Despite careful planning, unforeseen ethical dilemmas may still emerge. For instance, participants might inadvertently capture images of others without their consent, or their perspectives on sharing certain images may shift over time. In such situations, researchers must remain ethically reflexive by prioritising participants' well-being, safeguarding anonymity, and upholding legal and ethical standards, while also respecting participants' autonomy and lived experiences. By embedding these principles into the research design, researchers can promote more ethical, inclusive, and socially responsible photographic research practices.

7.2.2 Confidentiality and privacy

Researchers have a legal and moral duty to protect participants' personal data, ensuring compliance with legislative frameworks such as the GDPR and upholding participants' rights, including the right to a private life. In photography-based research, the potential for identifying individuals is heightened because photographs may contain recognisable faces, locations, or objects that can inadvertently reveal a participant's identity or circumstances. Moreover, digital photographs often carry embedded metadata such as GPS coordinates, device IDs, or usernames that can compromise confidentiality by disclosing sensitive information like a participant's home address or workplace. This issue is particularly critical when participants share images electronically via platforms like Google Photos®, OneDrive®, or iCloud®, which may also store and transmit metadata. To mitigate these risks, researchers can use metadata removal tools such as ExifCleaner® or MAT2® (Metadata Anonymisation Toolkit) to strip identifying information from digital photographs before storage or dissemination.

Similarly, wearable cameras introduce additional privacy concerns due to their capacity for continuous, passive recording of participants' environments. As Meyer et al. (2022) warn, these devices can inadvertently capture third parties, sensitive locations, or private moments without explicit consent, raising ethical questions about the scope of data collection and visibility of participants' daily lives. This introduces a further layer of ethical complexity, as researchers must also consider confidentiality and privacy rights of individuals who are not formally enrolled in the study but may appear in photographs or video footage.

In such cases, researchers should implement strategies to minimise third-party identification, such as image blurring, cropping, or obtaining retrospective consent where feasible, and address these risks explicitly in ethics applications and participant information materials. However, faces, gestures, and contextual cues often carry deep emotional resonance, allowing viewers to connect with the subject's experience on a human level. When these elements are obscured, the image may lose its capacity to evoke empathy or convey the full depth of the participants' narrative. Therefore, anonymisation risks shifting a photograph from a deeply personal artefact to a more abstract representation, potentially weakening its power. As a result, researchers must carefully weigh the ethical imperative of anonymity against the communicative intent of the image, and consider participant-led strategies that preserve meaning while safeguarding identity (Mannay, 2016).

To further safeguard privacy while preserving the expressive potential of photographic data, researchers can encourage participants to use indirect or symbolic imagery that conveys human experiences without revealing identifiable features. This may include photographing objects, environments, or textures that hold personal significance, or using visual metaphors, for example, a closed door to represent isolation or a doll to represent childhood experiences (Figure 7.1).

Participants might also capture partial body representations (e.g., hands, feet, silhouettes, or shadows) that evoke presence and emotion without disclosing identity. These strategies illustrated in Figures 7.2 and 7.3 allow for rich narrative expression while reducing the risk of disclosure.

Internal confidentiality or deductive disclosure is another key aspect to consider. It occurs when traits of individuals or groups make them identifiable in research reports (Kaiser, 2009). For example, during the COVID-19 pandemic, a healthcare worker participating in a visual diary study might submit a photograph of their PPE (Personal Protective Equipment) including identifiable contextual details such as a staff-only noticeboard, a ward number, or a distinctive uniform badge. In smaller hospitals or specialised units, these visual cues, combined with knowledge of the participant's role or shift patterns, could allow colleagues or community members to identify them. This highlights how confidentiality can be compromised through environmental and contextual elements within photographs, even in the absence of facial recognition.

To mitigate these risks, researchers must justify the collection and storage of personally identifiable information, including visual data. A robust data management strategy should be implemented, ensuring identifiable information (e.g., contact details, demographic data, healthcare records, and photographs) is stored separately from research data. Secure storage solutions such as password-protected devices, encrypted servers, and restricted-access facilities are essential to prevent unauthorised access.

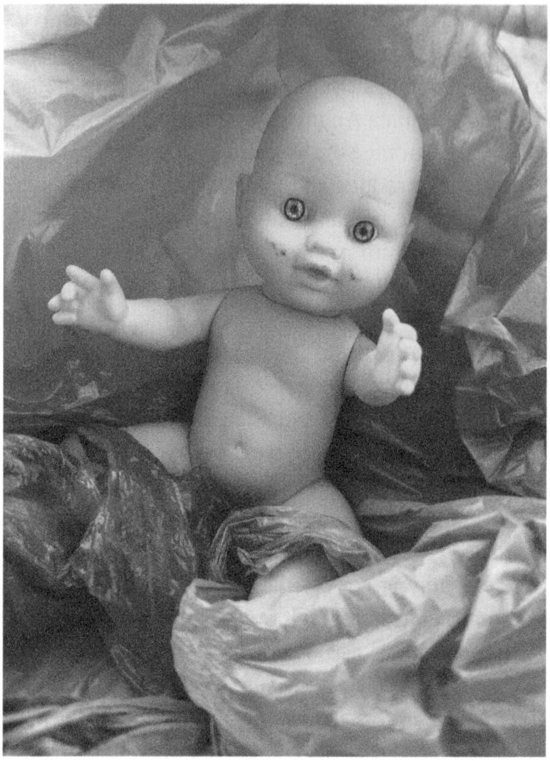

FIGURE 7.1 "Lost childhood"

Source: photograph by Laura

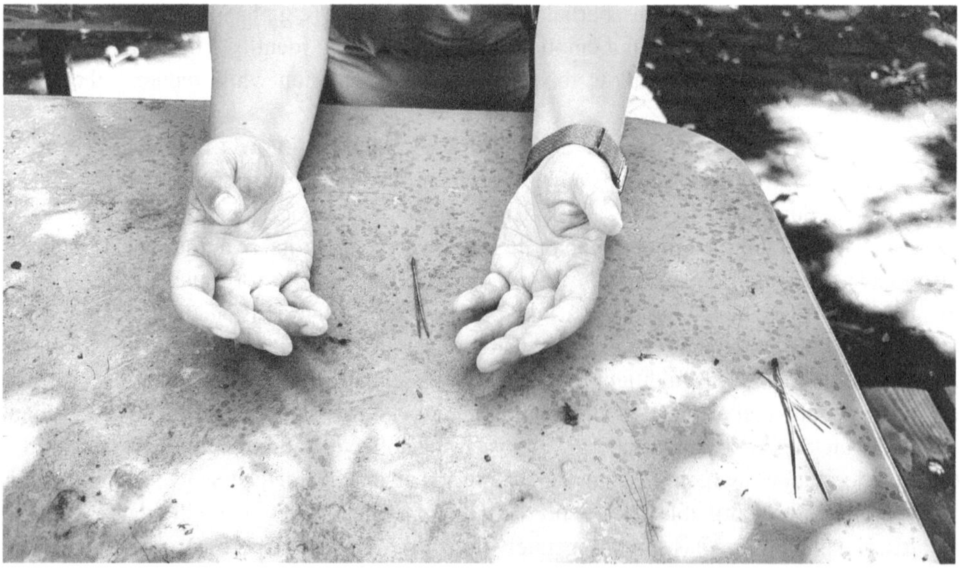

FIGURE 7.2: "I am here for you"

Source: photograph by Laura

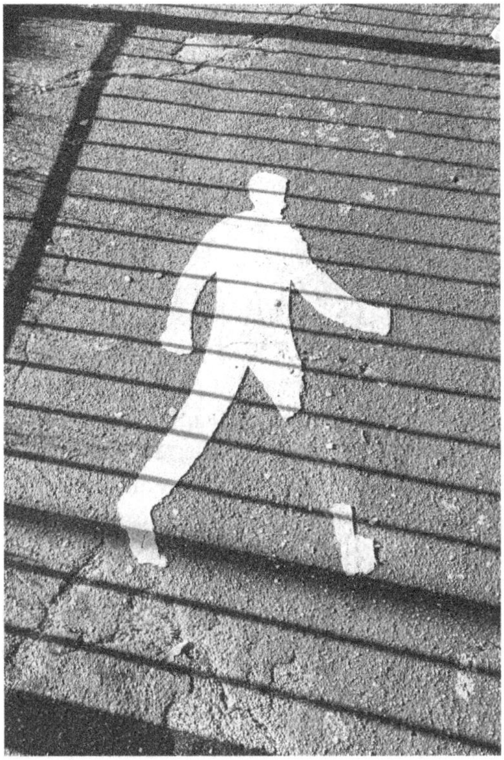

FIGURE 7.3 "Fractured self"

Source: photograph by the Author

Participants should be fully informed about how their verbal, textual, and visual data will be handled. Confidentiality agreements can outline the scope of data use, including the duration of storage, the nature of dissemination, and the specific conditions under which confidentiality may be breached. For instance, researchers are ethically and sometimes legally obligated to breach confidentiality if a participant discloses imminent harm to themselves or others, a risk that is particularly heightened in health research. Similarly, breaches of confidentiality may be justified in the public interest, such as when uncovering systemic injustices, unlawful practices, or professional misconduct in healthcare. These boundaries should be clearly communicated during the consent process and explicitly outlined in participant information sheets (Surmiak, 2018).

The format of photographic data also influences confidentiality considerations. While physical formats (e.g., polaroids, prints) pose risks of physical loss or unauthorised viewing, digital formats introduce challenges related to data transfer and storage. Email, for example, may be unsuitable due to attachment size limits and security vulnerabilities. Regardless of format, researchers should minimise the collection of identifiable information and adopt clear data management protocols for data handling.

Additional ethical tensions may arise in participatory and action-oriented research, where the goal is often to share participants' experiences publicly to drive social change. As Ponic and Jategaonkar (2012) and Reid and Brief (2009) note, broad dissemination, for example, in community venues, can reduce participant confidentiality and autonomy. This is particularly concerning in small communities or among vulnerable populations, such as women who have left abusive relationships, or individuals with HIV or other highly stigmatising conditions. Publicly displayed photographs may expose participants to stigma, retaliation, or social exclusion, especially if their identities or locations are recognisable.

This aspect of public dissemination often brings participatory research into tension with Institutional Review Boards (IRBs), which are typically structured around more traditional, individualised notions of risk and protection. As McDonald and Capous-Desyllas (2021) argue, IRBs may impose restrictions that conflict with the collaborative and emancipatory goals of community-based participatory research, particularly when participants wish to be acknowledged as authors of their photographs and have their visual narratives shared publicly. To navigate these tensions, researchers can engage in proactive dialogue with ethics committees, presenting context-specific justifications for participatory practices and considering flexible ethical frameworks that respect participants' self-determination. Involving participants in these discussions through advisory roles or co-authorship can further strengthen ethical transparency and help bridge the gap between institutional requirements and community-based research values. Bussu et al. (2021) claim that ethical engagement in participatory research must go beyond procedural compliance to embrace relational ethics, where trust, mutual respect, and shared decision-making are central. This requires researchers to challenge rigid institutional norms and advocate for ethical review processes that are responsive to the lived realities and priorities of participants, particularly in health-related contexts where vulnerability and power imbalances are often pronounced.

While confidentiality is not an absolute legal requirement, it remains a core professional and ethical responsibility. In photography-based health research, researchers must carefully balance the obligation to protect participants with the potential benefits of sharing visual narratives, always prioritising participants' safety, dignity, informed consent, transparency, and data security.

7.2.3 Anonymisation and pseudonymisation

Closely related to confidentiality, anonymisation and pseudonymisation are both data protection techniques used to safeguard personal information, but they differ significantly in their purpose, reversibility, and legal implications. More specifically, *anonymisation* refers to the process of irreversibly removing or altering personal identifiers so that individuals can no longer be identified, directly or indirectly. While anonymisation is permanent in nature, *pseudonymisation* is reversible, meaning that identities can be restored. This is because pseudonymisation consists of replacing or masking personal identifiers with artificial identifiers or pseudonyms, while retaining the ability to re-identify the data (Tinabo et al., 2009).

In the context of photography-based research, anonymisation may involve blurring or pixelating faces, removing metadata, or avoiding the inclusion of identifiable landmarks or objects. While these techniques can reduce the risk of identification, they are not foolproof. As Cleland and MacLeod (2021) note, even anonymised photographs may still be recognisable to individuals familiar with the context, such as local community members. Moreover, anonymisation in photographic research can be ethically complex. Blurring faces, for instance, may protect identity but can also objectify or dehumanise the subject, reducing the emotional impact and authenticity of the image (Allen, 2015).

In participatory research, ethical considerations around anonymisation and pseudonymisation are particularly complex, especially when visual narratives are central to participants' voices and agency (Wiles et al., 2011). Participants may view attribution not only as a matter of recognition but also as a form of empowerment and resistance to stigma (Giordano et al., 2007). For instance, in a study involving individuals in recovery from substance use (Smith et al., 2024), several participants explicitly requested to use their real names to promote transparency and raise awareness, leaving the researchers with a conundrum. While this aligns with the participatory ethos of amplifying marginalised voices, it also introduces ethical tensions. As a result, researchers must carefully balance respect for participants' autonomy with the responsibility to protect them from potential long-term harms, such as reputational damage or emotional distress.

This tension is further illustrated in Creighton et al.'s (2018a, 2018b) photovoice study on bereavement through male suicide, where participants chose to share portraits of family members or self-portraits. Although the research team initially hesitated due to concerns about informed consent and emotional vulnerability, they ultimately honoured the participants' decision, recognising that excluding the image would contradict the participatory principles of the project. However, researchers often opt not to publish participants' real names, even when requested, citing the potential for unforeseen consequences and tensions with Institutional Review Boards. Such decisions, while protective, can also be perceived as paternalistic and disempowering (Evans-Agnew & Rosemberg, 2016).

Ultimately, decisions about anonymisation and pseudonymisation should be made collaboratively with participants from the outset of the project. Researchers must clearly communicate the risks and limitations of each approach and ensure that participants' choices are informed, respected, and documented. As Smith et al. (2024) argues, these decisions should be defensible, context-sensitive, and grounded in a commitment to participant well-being, without undermining their agency or silencing their voices.

7.2.4 (Mis)representation

In photography-based health research, particularly within participatory methodologies such as photovoice, the ethics of representation are both complex and consequential. Photographs are powerful conveyors of meaning, yet their interpretation is never fixed. Clark-Ibáñez's (2007) reflected on this topic, concluding that the adage "photographs never lie" belies the reality that images are inherently open to multiple readings, shaped by the viewer's context, assumptions, and cultural frameworks. This ambiguity raises critical ethical questions about how images are produced, curated, edited, shared, and ultimately understood.

A central concern is the potential for misrepresentation, whether intentional or inadvertent. When researchers manipulate photographs through cropping, colour adjustment, or digital enhancement, there is a risk of distorting the participant's intended message or presenting a reality that aligns more closely with the researcher's narrative than the participant's lived experience. Such interventions not only introduce bias into the research but also risk eroding the trust underpinning participatory approaches and compromising data authenticity and integrity. For this reason, academic journals started including in their "Instructions for Authors" information about which types of digital manipulations are acceptable, and which are not, particularly relevant within the context of using AI to generate and edit images.

However, participant-led manipulation of their own photographs often observed in photovoice studies (Madrigal et al., 2014) opens up a different ethical terrain. When participants edit their images – whether to obscure identities, enhance symbolism, or express aspirational realities – these alterations become part of the data itself. Comparing original and edited versions can offer valuable insights into the participant's internal world, highlighting tensions between current realities and desired futures, for example. These visual modifications should not be seen as distortions but as meaning-making tools, offering insight into how individuals conceptualise their health narratives over time (Milasan, 2022). This interpretive layering enriches data rather than compromising it, provided participants retain control over the process.

The issue of anonymity further complicates representation. While digital tools such as pixelation or blurring can protect identities, they may also strip images of their emotional resonance or context, as pointed out previously. Banks (2019) argues that anonymisation techniques can inadvertently lead to misrepresentation by dehumanising subjects and reducing them to abstract figures rather than individuals with stories to tell. This tension underscores the need for participant-led decisions about image use and modification.

Consent and control over image dissemination are critical ethical considerations in photography-based research. As Smith et al. (2024) emphasises, participants must retain the right to decide how and where their images are shared. However, even with comprehensive consent procedures and technical safeguards in place, researchers cannot fully prevent the unauthorised copying, repurposing, or misuse of images, particularly in digital environments. Creighton et al. (2018b) recounts a case in which a participant's photograph, despite protective measures, was copied and used without permission in a documentary funding pitch, violating the original agreement between researcher and participant. This incident underscores the limitations of institutional protections and highlights the need for transparent, ongoing communication with participants about potential risks associated with public dissemination of visual data.

Moreover, once photographs are shared in public spaces such as online galleries or physical exhibitions, they often acquire an "authorless" quality. Detached from the immediate presence or voice of the participant, these images invite viewers to engage with them through their own lenses, potentially projecting interpretations that diverge from the participant's intended message. This interpretive openness, while sometimes generative, also carries the risk of misrepresentation, particularly when images are viewed without adequate context. To mitigate this, photovoice research frequently pairs photographs with participant-generated narratives or pieces of creative writing for example, poetry, which serve to anchor the viewer's understanding and preserve the integrity of the participant's voice (Andina-Díaz et al., 2023). Furthermore, developing visual literacy among both researchers and audiences can help mitigate misinterpretation. Rose (2016) claims that without this literacy, images are more likely to be misunderstood or stripped of their intended meaning, especially in research contexts involving sensitive or complex narratives. Training in how to read and contextualise images critically allows for a deeper engagement with visual data and reduces the risk of reductive or biased interpretations.

7.2.5 Power dynamics

Power dynamics are an inescapable feature of photography-based health research, particularly when working with vulnerable individuals or communities such as patients, children, older adults, inmates, or those from low-income or marginalised backgrounds. These dynamics shape not only the research process but also the ethics of representation, participation, and dissemination. While photography introduces additional ethical complexities, it also offers opportunities to democratise research by enabling participants to assert their voices and challenge dominant narratives (Sankey, 2014).

A critical distinction in ethical frameworks is that between *condescending* and *relational* ethics. *Relational* ethics, as articulated by Ponic and Jategaonkar (2012), emphasise mutual respect, dignity, and connectedness between researchers and participants. This approach recognises that ethical decisions are always situated within broader social, cultural, and political contexts. Rather than assuming a neutral or detached stance, relational ethics call for researchers to be reflexively aware of their own positionality and the power they hold in shaping the research agenda, interpretation, and outcomes (Phillips et al., 2021). In contrast, *condescending* ethics adopt a top-down approach, where researchers assume authority over participants' well-being, potentially silencing their voices and reinforcing power imbalances (Eikeland, 2006).

Clark et al. (2010) propose the concept of "situated visual ethics" as particularly appropriate for image-based research. This framework is a context-sensitive, participant-informed approach to consent, anonymity, and confidentiality. It recognises that ethical decisions cannot be standardised but must be co-constructed with participants in ways that respect their values, beliefs, and lived experiences.

In participatory methodologies like photovoice, power-sharing is not merely aspirational but foundational. Consequently, the researcher's role shifts from expert to facilitator of ongoing dialogue and reflection. Participants are encouraged to determine for themselves whether and how participation is safe and meaningful within the context of their lives (O'Sullivan et al., 2023). This approach requires a flexible, negotiated understanding of ethics that is responsive to participants' evolving needs and situated realities.

Despite these participatory intentions, photovoice research is not immune to reproducing oppressive power relations. As cautioned by Smith et al. (2024), asking participants to document their communities can become disempowering if it is not grounded in a genuine commitment to amplifying their voices and addressing issues that matter to them. Power imbalances rooted in differential access to resources, education, and institutional authority can never be fully eliminated. However, they must be acknowledged, discussed, and actively negotiated throughout the research process (Abma et al., 2022).

Communication in photovoice should not be framed as a unidirectional extraction of information by the researcher, but rather as a dialogical process of mutual learning and co-creation. This is particularly important when ethical tensions arise around image use. For example, excluding a participant's photograph from dissemination despite having obtained informed consent may contradict the core principles of photovoice, which aim to destigmatise sensitive issues and provide platforms for marginalised individuals to be seen and heard (Ng et al., 2023). In such cases, overprotective decisions by researchers or ethics boards may appear paternalistic, compromising the agency of participants and the emancipatory goals of the research (Creighton et al., 2018b).

Ultimately, ethical engagement with power dynamics in photography-based health research requires more than procedural compliance. It demands a sustained commitment to reflexivity, transparency, and shared decision-making. Researchers must reflect on, and develop awareness of, the ways in which their actions, assumptions, and institutional affiliations may shape the research encounter, and be willing to share control over the research process in favour of more equitable, participant-led practices.

7.2.6 Ownership and copyright

Ownership and copyright are central ethical considerations in photography-based health research, particularly in participatory approaches such as photovoice. In the United Kingdom, copyright law recognises the photographer as the legal owner of the image from the moment it is created, without the need for formal registration. Under the Copyright, Designs and Patents Act 1988 (as amended by the Intellectual Property Act 2014), this ownership typically lasts for the creator's lifetime plus 70 years. Therefore, when participants take photographs as part of a research project, they retain copyright unless they have explicitly transferred it or created the work in the course of employment.

This legal framework has important implications for research practice. Participants should be clearly informed that they own the rights to their images and should be given the opportunity to decide how their photographs are used, shared, and credited. Most photovoice projects respect this default legal position, ensuring participants receive personal copies of their images and are acknowledged as creators (Oakes et al., 2023). Researchers, in turn, are typically granted a licence through a consent agreement to use photographs for specific purposes such as analysis, publication, or exhibition. These agreements should be written in accessible language and include options for participants to define the scope of image use.

However, institutional policies may vary, and researchers must address potential tensions between participant ownership and university or funder requirements. Some institutions may seek broader rights over research outputs, including images, which can conflict with the participatory ethos of photovoice. It is therefore essential to clarify ownership and usage rights at the outset of the project and facilitate participant control wherever possible.

The digital nature of contemporary photography introduces further ethical complications. Once images are shared online or exhibited publicly, they can be copied, altered, or disseminated beyond the original scope of the research (Creighton et al., 2018b). This raises concerns about loss of control, especially when images are emotionally or politically charged. Researchers must acknowledge these risks and ensure that participants are fully aware of the potential for unintended circulation. As Smith et al. (2024) notes, sustaining participant ownership is not only a legal obligation but also an ethical commitment to protecting the integrity and intent of their visual narratives. Therefore, ethical image use in photography-based research must go beyond legal compliance to embrace a relational and participatory approach. This includes respecting copyright, ensuring informed and ongoing consent, and supporting participants in making decisions about the life of their images both within and beyond the research project.

Conclusion

Ethics in photography-based health research extends far beyond procedural compliance and a static checklist of ethical considerations. It is a dynamic, context-sensitive process that demands reflexivity, transparency, and respect for participant agency. While visual methods offer unique opportunities for empowerment, expression, and advocacy, they also introduce complex ethical challenges around autonomy, consent, confidentiality, representation, and ownership. These challenges are amplified in participatory research, where the tension between protecting participants and honouring their desire for visibility must be cautiously negotiated. Researchers must move beyond rigid frameworks toward relational and situated ethics, co-constructing decisions with participants and acknowledging the power dynamics inherent in visual inquiry. Practical strategies such as iterative consent, anonymisation balanced with narrative integrity, and participant-led dissemination, are essential for safeguarding dignity while preserving the expressive potential of photography.

Knowledge check

1. In what ways might participatory photography pose psychological risks to both participants and researchers, and what strategies can be implemented to mitigate such risks?
2. How can researchers ethically address the tension between protecting participant anonymity and honouring their desire for visibility and recognition in photography-based research?
3. Why is it important for researchers to reflect on their own positionality and authority in photographic research, and how might this influence the co-production of knowledge?
4. Give examples of how misrepresentation can occur in photography-based health research, and explain how researcher decisions such as editing, anonymisation, or selective dissemination might unintentionally distort participant narratives.

References

Abma, T., Breed, M., Lips, S., & Schrijver, J. (2022). Whose voice is it really? Ethics of photovoice with children in health promotion. *International Journal of Qualitative Methods, 21*(1), 1–11. https://doi.org/10.1177/16094069211072419

Allen, L. (2015). Losing face? Photo-anonymisation and visual research integrity. *Visual Studies, 30*(3), 295–308. https://doi.org/10.1080/1472586X.2015.1016741

Andina-Díaz, E., Siles-González, J., Gutiérrez-García, A. I., & Solano-Ruiz, M. C. (2023). Perception of care from the perspective of nursing students: A study using photovoice, storytelling and poetry. *Nurse Education in Practice, 72*(1), 103791. https://doi.org/10.1016/j.nepr.2023.103791

Banks, M. (2019). *Using visual data in qualitative research.* Sage Publications Ltd.

Barry, J., Monahan, C., Monahan, M., Murphy, R., Ferguson, S., Lee, K., Bennett, A., Gibbons, P., & Higgins, A. (2021). "The road we travel": Developing a co-produced narrative for a photovoice project. *Journal of Psychiatric and Mental Health Nursing, 28*(4), 632–643. https://doi.org/10.1111/jpm.12709

Beauchamp, T. L., & Childress, J. F. (1989). *Principles of biomedical ethics* (3rd ed.). Oxford University Press.

Bergum, V., & Dossetor, J. D. (2005). *Relational ethics: The full meaning of respect.* University Publishing Group.

Berti Suman, A. (2024). Behind the scenes: Unpacking approaches and impact. In A. Berti Suman (Ed.), *Civic monitoring for environmental law enforcement.* Edward Elgar Publishing.

Breny, J. M., & McMorrow, S. L. (2021). *Photovoice for social justice: Visual representation in action* (1st ed.). Sage Publications Ltd. https://doi.org/10.4135/9781071938966

Budig, K., Diez, J., Conde, P., Sastre, M., Hernán, M., & Franco, M. (2018). Photovoice and empowerment: Evaluating the transformative potential of a participatory action research project. *BMC Public Health, 18*(1), 1–9. https://doi.org/10.1186/s12889-018-5335-7

Bussu, S., Lalani, M., Pattison, S., & Marshall, M. (2021). Engaging with care: Ethical issues in participatory research. *Qualitative Research, 21*(5), 667–685. https://doi.org/10.1177/1468794120904883

Catalani, C., & Minkler, M. (2010). Photovoice: A review of the literature in health and public health. *Health Education & Behavior, 37*(3), 424–451. https://doi.org/10.1177/1090198109342084

Clark, A., Prosser, J., & Wiles, R. (2010). Ethical issues in image-based research. *Arts & Health, 2*(1), 81–93. https://doi.org/10.1080/17533010903495298

Clark-Ibáñez, M. (2007). "Inner-city children in sharper focus: Sociology of childhood and photo elicitation interviews". In G. C. Stanczak (Eds.), *Visual research methods: Image, society, and representation* (pp. 167–196). Sage Publications Ltd.

Cleland, J., & MacLeod, A. (2021). The visual vernacular: Embracing photographs in research. *Perspectives in Medical Education, 10*(4), 230–237. https://doi.org/10.1007/s40037-021-00672-x

Creighton, G., Oliffe, J. L., Bottorff, J., & Johnson, J. (2018a). "I should have . . .": A photovoice study with women who have lost a man to suicide. *American Journal of Men's Health, 12*(5), 1262–1274. https://doi.org/10.1177/1557988318760030

Creighton, G., Oliffe, J. L., Ferlatte, O., Bottorff, J., Broom, A., & Jenkins, E. K. (2018b). Photovoice ethics: Critical reflections from men's mental health research. *Qualitative Health Research, 28*(3), 446–455. https://doi.org/10.1177/1049732317729137

Edmondson, A. J., Brennan, C., & House, A. O. (2018). Using photo-elicitation to understand reasons for repeated self-harm: A qualitative study. *BMC Psychiatry, 18*(1), 1–11. https://doi.org/10.1186/s12888-018-1681-3

Eikeland, O. (2006). Condescending ethics and action research. *Action Research, 4*(1), 37–47. https://doi.org/10.1177/1476750306060541

Evans-Agnew, R. A., & Rosemberg, M. A. S. (2016). Questioning photovoice research: Whose voice? *Qualitative Health Research, 26*(8), 1019–1030. https://doi.org/10.1177/1049732315624223

Fahie, D. (2014). Doing sensitive research sensitively: Ethical and methodological issues in researching workplace bullying. *International Journal of Qualitative Methods, 13*(1), 19–36. https://doi.org/10.1177/160940691401300108

Florea, M. (2023). Withdrawal of consent for processing personal data in biomedical research. *International Data Privacy Law, 13*(2), 107–123. https://doi.org/10.1093/idpl/ipad008

Giordano, J., O'Reilly, M., Taylor, H., & Dogra, N. (2007). Confidentiality and autonomy: The challenge(s) of offering research participants a choice of disclosing their identity. *Qualitative Health Research, 17*(2), 264–275. https://doi.org/10.1177/1049732306297884

Groot, B. C., Schrijver, J., & Abma, T. A. (2021). Are you afraid of press and social media? Ethics in photovoice in participatory health research. *Educational Action Research, 31*(3), 556–574. https://doi.org/10.1080/09650792.2021.1941164

Hamilton, J., Ingham, B., McKinnon, I., Parr, J. R., Tam, L. Y.-C., & Le Couteur, A. (2017). Mental capacity to consent to research? Experiences of consenting adults with intellectual disabilities and/or autism to research. *British Journal of Learning Disabilities, 45*(4), 229–237. https://doi.org/10.1111/bld.12198

Kaiser, K. (2009). Protecting respondent confidentiality in qualitative research. *Qualitative Health Research, 19*(11), 1632–1641. https://doi.org/10.1177/1049732309350879

Klykken, F. H. (2021). Implementing continuous consent in qualitative research. *Qualitative Research, 22*(5), 795–810. https://doi.org/10.1177/14687941211014366

Kramer, L., Schwartz, P., Cheadle, A., Borton, J. E., Wright, M., Chase, C., & Lindley, C. (2010). Promoting policy and environmental change using photovoice in the Kaiser Permanente Community Health Initiative. *Health Promotion Practice, 11*(3), 332–339. https://doi.org/10.1177/1524839909341555

Langmann, S., & Pick, D. (2017). Ethical considerations in photography as a research method. In S. Langmann & D. Pick (Eds.), *Photography as a social research method* (pp. 57–83). Springer. https://doi.org/10.1007/978-981-10-7279-6_3

Madrigal, D. S., Salvatore, A., Casillas, G., Casillas, C., Vera, I., Eskenazi, B., & Minkler, M. (2014). Health in my community: Conducting and evaluating PhotoVoice as a tool to promote environmental health and leadership among Latino/a youth. *Progress in Community Health Partnerships: Research, Education, and Action, 8*(3), 317–329. https://doi.org/10.1353/cpr.2014.0034

Mannay, D. (2016). The politics of visibility, voice and anonymity: Ethically disseminating visual research findings without the pictures. In D. Warr, M. Guillemin, S. Cox, & J. Waycott (Eds.), *Ethics and visual research methods* (pp. 151–164). Palgrave Macmillan. https://doi.org/10.1057/978-1-137-54305-9_17

McDonald, L. E., & Capous-Desyllas, M. (2021). Navigating ethical issues in photovoice: Balancing the principles of community-based participatory research ethics with Institutional Review Board requirements. *Journal of Empirical Research on Human Research Ethics, 16*(4), 364–373. https://doi.org/10.1177/15562646211032777

Meyer, L. E., Porter, L., Reilly, M. E., Johnson, C., Safir, S., Greenfield, S. F., Silverman, B. C., Hudson, J. I., Javaras, K. N. (2022). Using wearable cameras to investigate health-related daily life experiences: A literature review of precautions and risks in empirical studies. *Research Ethics, 18*(1), 64–83. https://doi.org/10.1177/17470161211054021

Milasan, L. H. (2022). Photo-elicitation: Unleashing imagery in healthcare research. In K. Hinsliff-Smith, J. McGarry, & P. Ali (Eds.), *Arts based health care research: A multidisciplinary perspective* (pp. 51–67). Springer Nature Switzerland AG. https://doi.org/10.1007/978-3-030-94423-0_5

Milasan, L. H. (2023). "Mending fractured personalities": A photography-based cultural study of recovery from mental distress in Romania. *Transcultural Psychiatry, 60*(2), 226–243. https://doi.org/10.1177/13634615221119373

Moncur, W. (2013). The emotional wellbeing of researchers: Considerations for practice. In *Proceedings of the SIGCHI conference on human factors in computing systems* (pp. 1883–1890). Association for Computing Machinery. https://doi.org/10.1145/2470654.2466248

Ng, C. G., Ting, S. Q., Saifi, R. A., & Kamarulzaman, A. B. (2023). Ethical issues in photovoice studies involving key populations: A scoping review. *Asian Bioethics Review, 16*(1), 109–129. https://doi.org/10.1007/s41649-023-00264-3

Oakes, L. R., Ewald, D. R., Orsini, M. M., & Strack, R. W. (2023). The photovoice decision tree: Legal considerations and ethical implications for photographs and captions. *Health Promotion Practice, 24*(1), 123–132. https://doi.org/10.1177/15248399211053892

O'Sullivan, S., Desmond, E., & Buckley, M. (2023). The ethics of engagement and representation in community-based participatory research. *Ethics and Social Welfare, 17*(2), 159–174. https://doi.org/10.1080/17496535.2023.2211756

Phillips, L., Christensen-Strynø, M. B., & Frølunde, L. (2021). Thinking with autoethnography in collaborative research: A critical, reflexive approach to relational ethics. *Qualitative Research, 22*(5), 761–776. https://doi.org/10.1177/14687941211033446

Ponic, P., & Jategaonkar, N. (2012). Balancing safety and action: Ethical protocols for photovoice research with women who have experienced violence. *Arts & Health, 4*(3), 189–202. https://doi.org/10.1080/17533015.2011.584884

Reid, C., & Brief, E. (2009). Confronting condescending ethics: How community-based research challenges traditional approaches to consent, confidentiality, and capacity. *Journal of Academic Ethics, 7*(2–3), 75–85. https://doi.org/10.1007/s10805-009-9085-0

Roguljić, M., Šimunović, D., Buljan, I., Žuljević, M. F., Turić, A., & Marušić, A. (2025). Publishing identifiable patient photographs in the digital age: Focus group study of patients, doctors, and medical students. *Journal of Medical Internet Research, 27*(1), e59970. https://www.jmir.org/2025/1/e59970

Rose, G. (2016). *Visual methodologies: An introduction to researching with visual materials* (4th ed.). Sage Publications Ltd.

Saita, E., & Tramontano, M. (2018). Navigating the complexity of the therapeutic and clinical use of photography in psychosocial settings: A review of the literature. *Research in Psychotherapy: Psychopathology, Process and Outcome, 21*(1), 1–11. https://doi.org/10.4081/ripppo.2018.293

Sankey, M. D. (2014). From rags to riches: Democratisation of the photographic art. In V. Garnons-Williams (Ed.), *Photography & fictions: Locating dynamics of practice* (pp. 79–84). Queensland Centre for Photography.

Sanon, M. A., Evans-Agnew, R. A., & Boutain, D. M. (2014). An exploration of social justice intent in photovoice research studies from 2008 to 2013. *Nursing Inquiry, 21*(3), 212–226. https://doi.org/10.1111/nin.12064

Sherwin, S. (Ed.). (1998). *The politics of women's health: Exploring agency and autonomy*. Temple University Press.

Smith, B., Williams, O., Bone, L., & the Moving Social Work Collective (2022). Co-production: A resource to guide co-producing research in sport, exercise, and health sciences. *Qualitative Research in Sport, Exercise and Health, 15*(2), 159–187. https://doi.org/10.1080/2159676X.2022.2052946

Smith, E., Carter, M., Walklet, E., & Hazell, P. (2024). Exploring the methodological benefits and challenges of utilising a photovoice methodology with individuals in recovery from problem substance use. *Qualitative Health Research, 34*(10), 883–894. https://doi.org/10.1177/10497323231217601

Sontag, S. (1977). *On photography*. Farrar, Straus and Giroux.

Surmiak, A. D. (2018). Confidentiality in qualitative research involving vulnerable participants: Researchers' perspectives. *Forum: Qualitative Social Research, 19*(3), 1–26. https://doi.org/10.17169/fqs-19.3.3099

Teti, M. (2019). The murky ethics of visual qualitative methods: Picturing a clear path forward. *International Journal of Qualitative Methods, 18*(1), 1–4. https://doi.org/10.1177/1609406919884810

Tinabo, R., Mtenzi, F., & O'Shea, B. (2009). *Anonymisation vs. pseudonymisation: Which one is most useful for both privacy protection and usefulness of e-healthcare data*. IEEE. https://ieeexplore.ieee.org/document/5402501

Wiersma, E. C. (2011). Using photovoice with people with early-stage Alzheimer's disease: A discussion of methodology. *Dementia, 10*(2), 203–216. https://doi.org/10.1177/1471301211398990

Wiertz, S., & Boldt, J. (2022). Evaluating models of consent in changing health research environments. *Medicine, Health Care and Philosophy, 25*(2), 269–280. https://doi.org/10.1007/s11019-022-10074-3

Wiles, R., Coffey, A., Robinson, J., & Heath, S. (2011). Anonymisation and visual images: Issues of respect, 'voice' and protection. *International Journal of Social Research Methodology, 15*(1), 41–53. https://doi.org/10.1080/13645579.2011.564423

Xu, A., Baysari, M. T., Stocker, S. L., Day, R. O., & Carland, J. E. (2020). Researchers' views on, and experiences with, the requirement to obtain informed consent in research involving human participants: A qualitative study. *BMC Medical Ethics, 21*(1), 1–11. https://doi.org/10.1186/s12910-020-00538-7

8

PHOTOGRAPHY-BASED HEALTH RESEARCH IN THE ERA OF ARTIFICIAL INTELLIGENCE

8.1 AI and the death (or reimagining) of photography

Humanity has entered "hyperhistory" (Floridi, 2014) – a stage in human development where information has become the primary engine of progress, surpassing the dominance of manufacturing technologies. This era is marked by unprecedented global interconnectivity through vast flows of data. At the core of this transformation are algorithms or methods for extracting, generating, classifying, and predicting information that now shape the fabric of everyday life. Within this context, artificial intelligence (AI) technologies have been redefining how knowledge is produced, decisions are made, and social structures evolve. Their influence extends beyond technical domains, permeating aesthetic, ethical, and epistemological spheres, signalling a profound reconfiguration of human agency and creativity in an information-driven world.

The emergence of artificial intelligence within the photographic landscape has reignited longstanding anxieties about the survival of traditional media. Much like the 19th-century apprehension that photography would render painting obsolete, or the 20th-century fear that digital imaging would end analogue darkroom practices, today's discourse questions whether AI-generated imagery marks the death – or perhaps the radical reimagining – of photography itself. This debate, however, transcends simple binaries of "old" versus "new", "real" versus "fabricated". As Bateman and Hirsch (2025) observe, "truth in photography was never simple . . . from its earliest moments, photography has lived in tension between truth and art". The digital turn has already destabilised notions of photographic authenticity, while opening creative avenues for manipulation, abstraction, and surrealist expression (Tang & Misri, 2025).

Siri et al. (2022) describe photography's "changing identities" as a continual evolution – not only in its technological substrates, from film to digital to computational – but also in its cultural and aesthetic meanings. This evolution reflects not merely ontological shifts in what photography *is*, but perceptual shifts in how it is understood and experienced. Building on Don Idhe's (1995) framework and its recent adaptations to developments in the field of artificial intelligence (Wellner & Levin, 2024), post-phenomenology provides a useful philosophical lens that emphasises the mediating role of technology in shaping human experience. Photography, in this view,

DOI: 10.4324/9781003537540-9

is not a neutral recorder of reality but a dynamic interface that co-constitutes perception. Consequently, AI-generated images are not simply synthetic artifacts but new mediators of vision reshaping how we engage with the world, memory, and representation.

AI radically transforms the traditional object-subject relationship in photography by diluting its foundational link to reality. Classical photography is characterised by an indexical bond between image and object – a trace of light captured by a subject through a lens. This bond is grounded in the "referent" – the actual entity or scene that existed before the lens and left its imprint through light on a photosensitive surface. As Barthes (1981) famously argued, the photograph attests to the "that-has-been", anchoring its meaning in the ontological certainty of presence. In contrast, AI-generated imagery operates through algorithmic inference rather than physical presence, severing this ontological connection (Ballatore & Ballatore, 2024). As a result, the photographer's role as intentional agent is destabilised, with authorship becoming ambiguous, distributed across human prompts, algorithmic architectures, and vast datasets. This shift introduces profound confusion – if the image no longer records a real object, can it still be called a photograph? Post-phenomenological perspectives mentioned earlier help illuminate this regime of synthetic vision in which photography becomes less about capturing reality and more about generating possibilities of representation, imagination, and meaning – transforming the medium from an index of the real into a speculative interface for visual culture.

Without doubt, AI will continue to challenge the boundaries of the photographic medium, inviting us to reconsider what counts as photography and why. Schofield's (2024) notion of "media hauntology", suggesting that new media are always haunted by the spectres of prior forms, may help with exploring this terrain. In this light, even AI-generated images carry the ghostly imprint of photographic tradition. The dematerialisation of photography from physical print to digital code to algorithmic prompt does not necessarily signify its disappearance, but rather its spectral persistence and reinvention. Photography, therefore, may not be dying as many of us fear; it is mutating into a hybrid practice that challenges inherited assumptions about vision, reality, and representation.

8.2 Advancing photography-based research with AI technologies

As illustrated in the previous section, the concept and practice of photography have undergone profound transformations following the evolution of AI technologies increasingly prevalent in day-to-day life. Breakthroughs in this area have been enhancing the accessibility of photographic techniques and expanding the creative capabilities of photographers (Chen, 2024). AI-powered photo editing and design software are widely accessible through smartphones and other digital devices requiring minimal expertise. Unwanted distractions in the photographs can be erased instantly, backgrounds can be removed or changed effortlessly, and gaps filled in a way that makes it difficult to trace artificial additions to the original photograph. The process is facilitated by conversational agents allowing users to describe the desired changes in a chat or conversational panel with prompts that make the process highly interactive and customisable (Upadhye, 2024).

AI capabilities to process photographs go far beyond the digital manipulation of images, consisting of adjusting colour balance or colourising black-and-white pictures, optimising the contrast, exposure, brightness, sharpness, resolution, and noise removal. AI can "see" images and "understand" them through computer vision technologies – a field of AI focused on enabling machines to interpret and understand visual information from the world, such as images and videos (Chavez & Blanke, 2021). In brief, AI algorithms can identify and interpret elements in a photograph such as faces, objects, or even scenes, which makes the process of intelligent retouching more effective often in batches of hundreds or thousands of pictures at once. Moreover, photographs or elements in a photograph can be categorised according to content or tags following specific user instructions, which is ideal for visual analysis in research. This is because AI can handle large datasets, perform complex tasks of visual analysis and categorisation, and identify trends much faster compared to conventional methods.

AI algorithms can also process text from images, including handwritten notes, and analyse it or even recognise facial emotions and extract demographic data from photographs. Additionally, image segmentation helps with isolating specific visual elements to facilitate detailed analysis and interpretation by visual researchers or, conversely, filtering out content deemed as irrelevant. As a result, AI-powered tools can create intuitive mapping and representation of data, making it easier for researchers to interpret and communicate the visual findings, and triangulate them with textual datasets (Ye et al., 2024).

Guinibert (2022) discusses applications such as GPT-4® and Google Cloud Vision® that have been revolutionising the thematic analysis of visual datasets and provide a more efficient, scalable, comprehensive, and cost-effective alternative to traditional methods like manual coding of photographs while maintaining the richness of insight. Augmented Reality (AR) takes this process a step further, allowing visual researchers to literally immerse themselves in data, for example, 3D models or animated photographs, and experience them creatively and interactively in a way that may benefit their understanding and interpretation (Hitch, 2023). Recent developments in Generative Adversarial Networks (GANs), that is, a subfield of "machine learning" or "deep learning" (Aggarwal et al., 2023) go beyond processing and analysing existing photographs. They open avenues for creating hyperrealistic but also surreal and dreamlike images from text descriptions interpreted through natural language processing or other images, and even converting them into artwork or vice versa. DALL-E 4®, Mid Journey®, Microsoft Designer®, Google Gemini®, and Canva® are only a few examples of applications highly popular for visual content creation with variable human input.

These advancements inevitably challenge the traditional understanding of photographs as mere imprints of light reflected from objects. Photographic creative processes and their authenticity are also questioned alongside the fundamental nature of what is considered real in a photograph. This is not only because of the immateriality of photographs as digital artefacts but also because of the widespread concept of "deepfakes" or fabricated images leading to scepticism, controversies, and an overall negative reputation, especially when AI is utilised for manipulating images for misinformation purposes (Hausken, 2024).

While AI-generated imagery is not an objective and truthful depiction of reality, this does not mean that it does not have any value in research. On the contrary, AI-generated images show significant potential in enhancing mental health research, for example. They offer new ways to explore and understand complex emotional and psychological states, providing both researchers and participants with innovative tools for expression and analysis (Milasan, 2024), similar to its application in psychotherapeutic practice (Milasan, 2026 – in press). Furthermore, GenAI facilitates co-production between AI and researchers and/or research participants by providing them with creative for emotional expression utilising diverse styles and techniques known as computational aesthetics (Bo et al., 2018).

Such tools, illustrated in Figure 8.1, can be adapted to enhance accessibility and personalisation of the creative act for individuals with limited creative skills, light sensitivity, mobility issues, and even visual impairments through speech-to-image or image-to-speech interfaces (Milasan, 2024). Techniques like natural language processing can also identify and correct language, making the process accessible for people with cognitive impairments, for example, dementia, or severe mental health problems in line with their needs and preferences (Le Glaz et al., 2021).

Considering such advantages, AI tools have the potential to profoundly influence visual research and make it more engaging, flexible, and inclusive in ways that are not possible through conventional methods. These benefits are mediated by the way in which AI imagery is perceived. Grassini and Koivisto (2024) explored potential bias toward AI-generated art and found an intriguing paradox. Participants generally preferred AI-generated images and reported stronger positive emotions when the source was known, suggesting that AI imagery has achieved a high level of realism and emotional resonance. Yet, images perceived as AI-made, regardless of their

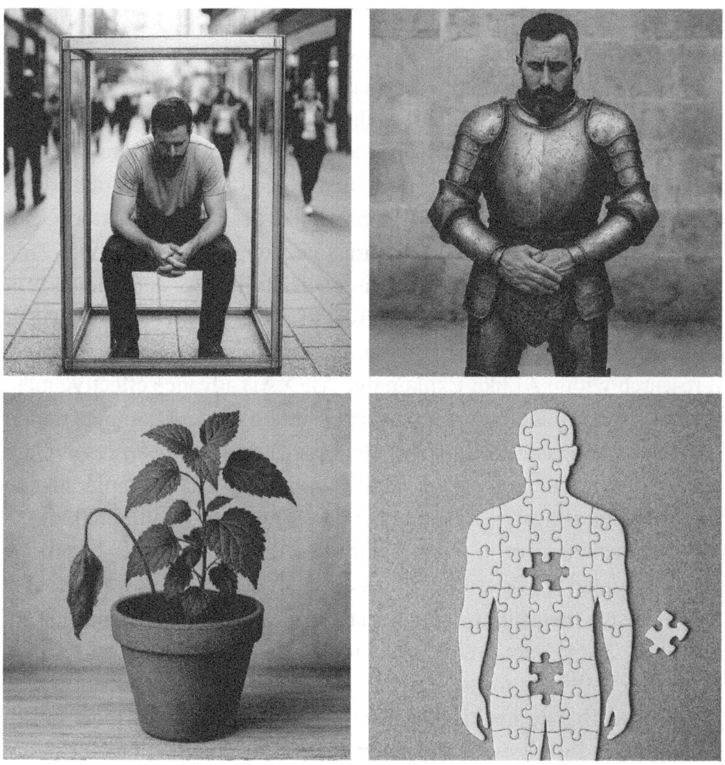

FIGURE 8.1 Visual metaphors generated with Copilot® to illustrate issues surrounding men's sexual health (top-left corner – Isolation, stigma, and silence; top-right corner – Vulnerability hidden behind societal expectations of masculinity; bottom-left corner – Erectile dysfunction; bottom-right corner – Self, identity, and sexual health). Prompt: "generate four hyperrealistic images to illustrate issues related to sexual health in men. Please use visual metaphors not explicit content".

actual origin, were rated more negatively. This indicates that perception, rather than intrinsic quality, strongly shapes attitudes toward AI imagery.

8.3 Ethical and methodological challenges related to using AI in photography-based research

Alongside the advantages of AI applications in photography-based research, literature also raises several ethical and methodological concerns. These issues are particularly pronounced in health research, which often involves highly sensitive data such as personal information and medical history that might be captured in photographs and patient narratives, for example. For this reason, researchers must be transparent about the use and storage of images, verbal, and textual contributions of research participants, and disclose if research data are shared with third parties, including AI software providers. Measures put in place such as anonymisation or pseudonymisation should be made clear, along with other actions to maintain confidentiality and protect privacy. This transparency is essential for building trust and ensuring that participants are fully informed about how AI is used to handle or interpret data. Prior to utilising AI software for research purposes, researchers must seek advice from experts to ensure compliance with data protection regulations and implement robust security measures. This is because AI systems and the data they rely on are vulnerable to cyberattacks and data breaches, potentially exposing sensitive information (National Institute of Standards and Technology, 2024).

However, the integration of AI in research and the principle of transparency often present significant challenges stemming from the complexity and opacity of AI algorithms, commonly referred to as the "black box" of AI. Some AI subsets, like deep learning models, can be extremely difficult to understand and explain hindering transparency and accountability in research practices (McCradden et al., 2020). Transparency in decision-making is particularly relevant in the context of informing patients and healthcare providers about how AI algorithms process data and why they make certain decisions and recommendations. This aspect continues to be problematic until fields of research within AI like Explainable AI (XAI) advance effective methods to bridge the gap between AI systems and human comprehension to make AI outputs understandable and explainable to humans (Ali et al., 2023). This can be an arduous task for researchers, particularly within the context of constantly evolving legal frameworks and the rapid advancements in AI applications across the healthcare sector and beyond (Zaidan & Ibrahim, 2024).

Another major ethical concern in photography-based and other types of research integrating AI solutions is represented by algorithmic bias and fairness. It is known that AI algorithms are trained on large datasets that might contain biases related to race, gender, or socio-economic status (Esposito et al., 2023; García-Ull & Melero-Lázaro, 2023; Nazer et al., 2023; Park, 2024). Ethically, this poses challenges to the fundamental principle of justice and fair representation due to the risk of exacerbating health disparities, if not implemented thoughtfully. The risk of perpetuating such biases by AI systems can have profound implications for the research methodology. For example, relying on AI-powered decision-making to select research participants can induce flaws, although there is evidence that AI can optimise the recruitment process in clinical trials (Lu et al., 2024). Subsequently, AI biases in recruitment can hinder demographic diversity with an impact on data collection, that might not be reflective of the perspectives of under-represented groups.

It is claimed that human validation at all research stages can help with improving methodological rigour and ensure ethical practices in research (Albassam, 2023). Literature debating whether researchers will be replaced by AI in the foreseeable future conclude that is highly unlikely considering activities that require semantic understanding such as research problem identification, theory building, and nuanced understanding of data that are currently areas in which AI does not excel (Kankanhalli, 2020). This applies to photography-based research in which interpretation of visual data may pose challenges to AI algorithms in terms of contextual understanding, exploring metaphorical and abstract images, and elucidating subtle cues in photographs as opposed to explicit features, which can lead to misinterpretations. In other words, AI is effective in recognising patterns in data, but is limited in its ability to "understand" meanings and contexts behind the photographs in the way humans do.

When AI is employed, researchers must be transparent about its limitations and declare them as part of the research outputs, for example, journal publications, alongside methods used for detecting and mitigating bias. While AI is unlikely to replace researchers in the foreseeable future, it remains an ideal assistant for researchers by completing automated tasks and processing large amounts of visual data that do not require critical thinking and creativity. However, AI capabilities evolve at a rapid pace, and ongoing advancements may gradually enhance its ability to interpret complex visual information and provide more insightful outcomes.

Conclusion

AI is reshaping the very concept of photography, which will undoubtedly have a major impact on visual research. By breaking its traditional link to reality and introducing synthetic vision, AI shifts photography from recording the real to generating new possibilities for expression and creativity. In photography-based health research, this transformation offers significant benefits, including greater accessibility, inclusivity, and creative potential. At the same time, it raises important ethical and methodological challenges around transparency, bias, and trust. The future of photography in health research will depend on how we balance these opportunities with critical reflection, ensuring that AI acts as a collaborator rather than a source of distortion or distraction. Rather than speculating on the fate of photography, we must consider how its evolving forms can continue to serve as meaningful instruments for inquiry and expression, enhancing the value of photography-based research.

Knowledge check

1. What are the methodological benefits and limitations of using AI in photography-based research?
2. What are the ethical implications of using AI in photography-based research, and how can they be addressed by researchers?

References

Aggarwal, A., Singh, N., & Parashar, S. K. (2023). Recent developments in generative adversarial networks. In *Artificial intelligence and sustainable computing* (pp. 163–172). Springer. https://doi.org/10.1007/978-981-99-1431-9_13

Albassam, A. W. (2023). The power of artificial intelligence in recruitment: An analytical review of current AI-based recruitment strategies. *International Journal of Professional Business Review, 8*(6), e02089. https://doi.org/10.26668/businessreview/2023.v8i6.2089

Ali, S., Abuhmed, T., El-Sappagh, S., Muhammad, K., Alonso-Moral, J. M., Confalonieri, R., Guidotti, R., Del Ser, J., Díaz-Rodríguez, N., & Herrera, F. (2023). Explainable artificial intelligence (XAI): What

we know and what is left to attain trustworthy artificial intelligence. *Information Fusion, 99*, 1–52. https://doi.org/10.1016/j.inffus.2023.101805
Ballatore, A., & Ballatore, F. (2024). Artificial "intelligence" and the ontology of art: A phenomenological inquiry. *Itinera, 28*(1), 118–129. https://doi.org/10.54103/2039-9251/27838
Barthes, R. (1981). *Camera Lucida: Reflections on photography*. Hill and Wang.
Bateman, E., & Hirsch, R. (2025). AI and the death of photography. *Journal of Images and Culture* [online]. https://vjic.org/vjic2/?page_id=8705
Bo, Y., Yu, J., & Zhang, K. (2018). Computational aesthetics and applications. *Visual Computing for Industry, Biomedicine, and Art, 1*, 6. https://doi.org/10.1186/s42492-018-0006-1
Chavez, D., & Blanke, T. (2021). On machine vision and photographic imagination. *AI & Society, 36*(4), 1–13. https://doi.org/10.1007/s00146-020-01091-y
Chen, Y. (2024). Artificial intelligence technology in photography and future challenges and reflections. *The Frontiers of Society, Science and Technology, 6*(6), 24–30. https://doi.org/10.25236/FSST.2024.060605
Esposito, P., Atighehchian, P., Germanidis, A., & Ghadiyaram, D. (2023). Mitigating stereotypical biases in text-to-image generative systems. *arXiv*. https://arxiv.org/abs/2310.06904
Floridi, L. (2014). *The fourth revolution: How the infosphere is reshaping human reality*. Oxford University Press.
García-Ull, F.-J., & Melero-Lázaro, M. (2023). Gender stereotypes in AI-generated images. *Profesional de la información, 32*(5), e320505. https://doi.org/10.3145/epi.2023.sep.05
Grassini, S., & Koivisto, M. (2024). Understanding how personality traits, experiences, and attitudes shape negative bias toward AI-generated artworks. *Scientific Reports, 14*(1), 1–15. https://doi.org/10.1038/s41598-024-54294-4
Guinibert, M. (2022). Computer-assisted qualitative visual analysis: Automating thematic analysis of images. *Interactions: Studies in Communication & Culture, 13*(The Human and the Machine: AI in Creative Industries), 147–167. https://doi.org/10.1386/iscc_00058_1
Hausken, L. (2024). Photorealism versus photography: AI-generated depiction in the age of visual disinformation. *Journal of Aesthetics & Culture, 16*(1), 1–13. https://doi.org/10.1080/20004214.2024.2340787
Hitch, D. (2023). Artificial intelligence augmented qualitative analysis: The way of the future? *Qualitative Health Research, 34*(7), 595–606. https://doi.org/10.1177/10497323231217392
Idhe, D. (1995). *Postphenomenology: Essays in the postmodern context*. Northwestern University Press.
Kankanhalli, A. (2020). Artificial intelligence and the role of researchers: Can it replace us? *Drying Technology, 38*(12), 1539–1541. https://doi.org/10.1080/07373937.2020.1801562
Le Glaz, A., Haralambous, Y., Kim-Dufor, D. H., Lenca, P., Billot, R., Ryan, T. C., Marsh, J., DeVylder, J., Walter, M., Berrouiguet, S., & Lemey, C. (2021). Machine learning and natural language processing in mental health: Systematic review. *Journal of Medical Internet Research, 23*(5), e15708. https://doi.org/10.2196/15708
Lu, X., Yang, C., Liang, L., Hu, G., Zhong, Z., & Jiang, Z. (2024). Artificial intelligence for optimizing recruitment and retention in clinical trials: A scoping review. *Journal of the American Medical Informatics Association, 31*(11), 2749–2759. https://doi.org/10.1093/jamia/ocae243
McCradden, M. D., Anderson, J. A., & Zlotnik Shaul, R. (2020). Accountability in the machine learning pipeline: The critical role of research ethics oversight. *The American Journal of Bioethics, 20*(11), 40–42. https://doi.org/10.1080/15265161.2020.1820111
Milasan, L. H. (2024). Unveiling the transformative potential of AI-generated imagery in enriching mental health research. *Qualitative Health Research* [e-pub]. https://doi.org/10.1177/10497323241274767
Milasan, L. H. (2026). Phototherapy, therapeutic photography and AI. In D. Lowenthal (Ed.), *Phototherapy and therapeutic photography in a digital age*. Routledge.
National Institute of Standards and Technology. (2024, January 4). *NIST identifies types of cyberattacks that manipulate behavior of AI systems*. https://www.nist.gov/news-events/news/2024/01/nist-identifies-types-cyberattacks-manipulate-behavior-ai-systems
Nazer, L. H., Zatarah, R., Waldrip, S., Ke, J. X. C., Moukheiber, M., Khanna, A. K., Hicklen, R. S., Moukheiber, L., Moukheiber, D., Ma, H., & Mathur, P. (2023). Bias in artificial intelligence algorithms and recommendations for mitigation. *PLOS Digital Health, 2*(6), e0000278. https://doi.org/10.1371/journal.pdig.0000278
Park, Y. S. (2024). White default: Examining racialized biases behind AI-generated images. *Art Education, 77*(4), 36–45. https://doi.org/10.1080/00043125.2024.2330340

Schofield, M. P. (2024). Camera Phantasma: Reframing virtual photographies in the age of AI. *Convergence: The International Journal of Research into New Media Technologies, 30*(2), 687–709. https://doi.org/10.1177/13548565231220314

Siri, H., Khairani, M. Z., & Halim, H. B. (2022). Digital photography and the future of photography culture. *International Journal of Applied and Creative Arts, 5*(1), 13–22. https://doi.org/10.33736/ijaca.4664.2022

Tang, Y., & Misri, I. B. (2025). Exploring surrealist approaches in digital media art for enhancing graphic and visual communication design. *Journal of Humanities Music and Dance, 5*(51), 1–14. https://doi.org/10.55529/jhmd.51.1.14

Upadhye, S. (2024). AI in image editing and enhancement: Revolutionizing photography. *International Journal of Modern Engineering & Management Research, 12*(2), 5–12. https://www.ijmemr.org/Publication/V12I2/IJMEMR-V12I2-001.pdf

Wellner, G., & Levin, I. (2024). Ihde meets Papert: Combining postphenomenology and constructionism for a future agenda of philosophy of education in the era of digital technologies. *Learning, Media and Technology, 49*(4), 656–669. https://doi.org/10.1080/17439884.2023.2251388

Ye, Y., Hao, J., Hou, Y., Wang, Z., Xiao, S., Luo, Y., & Zeng, W. (2024). Generative AI for visualization: State of the art and future directions. *Visual Informatics, 8*(2), 43–66. https://doi.org/10.1016/j.visinf.2024.04.003

Zaidan, E., & Ibrahim, I. A. (2024). AI governance in a complex and rapidly changing regulatory landscape: A global perspective. *Humanities and Social Sciences Communications, 11*, 1–12. https://doi.org/10.1057/s41599-024-03560-x

Further reading

Ritchin, F. (2025). *The synthetic eye: Photography transformed in the age of AI.* Thames & Hudson.

9

APPLICATIONS AND IDEAS FOR PHOTOGRAPHY-BASED RESEARCH ACTIVITIES IN HEALTHCARE

9.1 Applications

9.1.1 Reflection on the rationale for using photography in healthcare research (based on the content covered in Chapter 1)

You have been tasked with conducting a piece of research entitled "Capturing healing: a phenomenological study of post-surgery recovery through photography". As suggested by the title, this study aims to explore the experiences of patients recovering from major surgery by using photography as a research tool (and potentially a therapeutic method). In other words, participants will be asked to document their recovery journey through photographs, capturing moments meaningful to their physical, emotional, and mental states during the healing process.

Building on your knowledge developed throughout Chapter 1, complete the following tasks:

- Discuss how photography as a research method could enhance the phenomenological nature of this study.
- Explain how photography can become a therapeutic tool or a hindrance during the research process.
- Think about how a group versus individual approach to using photography as a research method would impact on the outcome of this study. Identify at least two benefits and two challenges to group and individual approaches.

9.1.2 Choosing the appropriate photographic technique in research (based on the content covered in Chapter 2)

A research student asks your advice on which photographic technique(s) would be most suitable for a study aiming to explore the journey toward recovery of individuals with testicular cancer: photo-elicitation, photovoice, photo-storytelling, or self-portraiture?

DOI: 10.4324/9781003537540-10

- Try to justify your suggestion by drawing on the knowledge provided in Chapter 2 regarding the benefits of each method in relation to the research topic.
- Can you think of any methodological drawbacks and challenges using any of the above photographic methods in researching such a sensitive subject?

9.1.3 *Formulating the research question (based on the content covered in Chapter 3)*

Critically appraise the following research question proposed by a healthcare research student for their dissertation from the point of view of structure, clarity, and feasibility:

> "How does participating in weekly photography-based workshops affect the emotional well-being of individuals experiencing pain over six months?"

Helping questions:

- Does the research question use the elements of a structured framework (e.g., PICO, PIO, SPIDER, etc.)?
- Can any of the key terms in the research question be made more specific, measurable, and actionable?
- How feasible is the research question from the point of view of population accessibility and intervention practicality?

9.1.4 *From research question to design (based on the content covered in Chapter 3)*

You identified your topic for a photography-based study looking at the role of photo-based food journaling (Intervention/I) in enhancing dietary adherence and perceived wellness (Outcomes/O) in young people with diabetes (Population/P).

- Think about different ways in which you could develop this study by implementing a range of sampling/recruitment strategies and sample sizes while considering pros and cons for each scenario.
- Reflect on how these choices might influence your study design and outcomes.

9.1.5 *Designing an interview guide for a photo-elicitation study (based on content covered in Chapter 4)*

Design a photo-elicitation semi-structured interview guide using 1. SHOWED, and 2. IMPARTED mnemonics for a photography-based study in your area of interest. Alternatively, use the scenario below to practice your skills to generate interview questions that could help you guide a photo-elicitation interview.

Title: "Exploring patient experiences in chronic illness management"
Aim: To understand the lived experiences of patients managing chronic illnesses (e.g., diabetes, heart disease) and identify challenges and facilitators in their daily care routines.

Photo assignment: Participants were asked to take photographs over a week depicting moments that reflect their experiences of managing their illness. These might include medication routines, meal preparations, exercise or mobility challenges, social interactions, and emotional highs and lows.

9.1.6 Designing a focus group guide for a photo-elicitation study (based on content covered in Chapter 4)

Generate a set of five questions to guide the facilitation of a photovoice group for a study exploring health inequities experienced by women living with endometriosis. The aim of this study is to examine and address systemic barriers affecting women with endometriosis in underserved communities by engaging participants and stakeholders in a collaborative effort to reduce health disparities in this area.

9.1.7 Data analysis (based on content covered in Chapter 5)

You are given Figure 9.1 alongside excerpts from a photo-elicitation interview within a study exploring lived experiences of caring for people with dementia (Table 9.1). This is a photograph I took specifically for this exercise, but the interview excerpts are fictional for educational purposes.

Your task is to analyse the photograph employing the 5Cs approach exemplified in Chapter 5 (Table 5.1) and triangulate different visual elements with the textual data in Table 9.1, while focusing on the transition from descriptive to interpretative visual analysis.

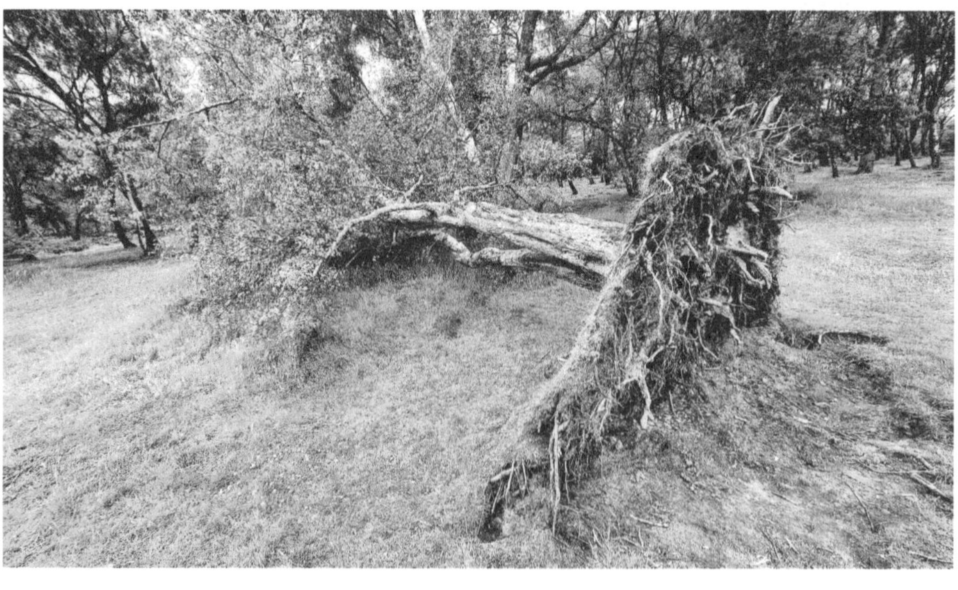

FIGURE 9.1 Uprooted tree

Source: photograph by the Author

TABLE 9.1 Excerpt from a fictional interview with a carer of a person living with dementia

Researcher (R): Could you please tell me what you tried to capture in this photograph?

Interviewee (I): I took this picture a couple of days ago in a park fifteen-minute drive from my home. Our home, I should say – my husband's as well, although it feels like he left a while ago, once his dementia got worse. He is still there though, hanging on, like this uprooted tree here [laughs with some unhappy undertones]. It happens that this is one of our favourite places probably because we used to date there in our green years [sighs]. We still go there at least once a week, although he [my husband] might not even recognise the place and all the memories we built there. . . There is a bench where we used to sit taking in the landscape for hours, reading a book or just chatting. I wouldn't trust him wonder around there on his own anymore though. . . Sorry, I am diverting here . . . What else shall I tell you?

R: You hinted at a comparison between this uprooted tree and your husband. Could you please tell me more what you had in mind when you said that?

I: I think so . . . Well . . . It [the comparison] came out of nowhere, to be honest. I didn't think about it until I looked closer at this picture. Well, to start with, I believe this tree might be my husband's age [laughs]. David [pseudonym] has also been through a lot of storms in his life, like us all. But he stood tall in front of all the challenges, like the other tree there in the background. And that's what kept me going. His strength and resilience that gave me a strong sense of security. But the last hurdle, I mean his dementia getting worse to the point that he often does not recognise me anymore, was a little too much . . . for both of us. It was a bit like the storm or the wind or whatever uprooted this tree in the picture . . . That's it, basically . . .

R: And how does that make you feel?

I: Well, sad, of course. Just seeing him defeated like that makes me sad. And worried, because I know there is no way back. I honestly do not think that he's going to get any better. And I also feel hopeless sometimes. I know that all the love and support I give him will not bring him back to what he used to be, what we used to be [starts sobbing].

R: I see that this conversation made you upset. Here is a tissue for you. . . I just want to remind you that we can always cut the interview short if this is too difficult for you to talk about.

I: No problems. On the contrary, it helps letting go some thoughts. One second [blows her nose]. I kind of lost the track of what I was saying. . .

R: No worries. Take your time. . . Let's see if there is anything else in the picture you took that might spark some ideas about your experience of caring for David [pseudonym].

I: I don't know if that was intentional or not, but I focused the camera on that messy tangle of roots that contrasts with all the natural beauty and the greenery around. . . Life is full of contrasts, isn't it? Sometimes it is a matter of perspective, of how you look at things. . . Take those roots, for example. Most likely, some of them are dead, rotten. . . It makes me think about neurons or synapses for some reason. . . Neurons that die with age, with illness like dementia, disconnected, kaput. . . You never know how many memories are left there buried in the ground that keep that tree alive despite it being knocked down. You can only hope there is something left you can nurture with hope and patience.

R: That is very profound. Thanks for sharing this.

9.1.8 Developing a dissemination plan (based on content covered in Chapter 6)

Develop a dissemination plan for the participatory photography-based research project outlined below and critically reflect on the strengths and limitations of various dissemination methods.

Title: "Through our eyes: Young adults' experiences of mental health recovery"

Description: In this project, participants aged 18–25 use photography to document and reflect on their personal journeys through mental health recovery. The aim is to explore how visual storytelling can challenge stigma, promote empathy, and inform service improvement.

Your task is to develop a dissemination plan that includes at least three different methods for sharing the findings. Consider a mix of academic (e.g., journal articles, conference presentations), community-based (e.g., exhibitions, photobooks, storyboards), and digital (e.g., social media, online galleries, virtual reality) strategies.

For each method:

- describe the target audience, the format (platform), and the intended impact or outcome.
- write a short reflection (100–150 words) focused on the advantages of your chosen dissemination methods, such as accessibility and engagement, and disadvantages or challenges, if any.

9.1.9 Ethical considerations (based on content covered in Chapter 7)

Imagine you are member of a Research Ethics Committee/Institutional Review Board and are asked to review an ethical application including the participant information sheet in Table 9.2. Read it carefully and answer the following questions:

- What ethical concerns can you identify in the participant information sheet provided?
- Which ethical principles (autonomy, non-maleficence, beneficence, and justice) are problematic, and why?
- What are your recommendations for addressing the ethical concerns you identified in the participant information sheet?

TABLE 9.2 Example of participant information sheet

PARTICIPANT INFORMATION SHEET
Research Project: Visual narratives of patient experiences in chronic illness management
Researcher: John Doe
What is this project about?
This research project explores patient experiences in managing chronic illnesses through the use of photography as a research method. The aim is to generate insights that can inform and enhance patient-centred care and support systems. My name is John Doe, and I am conducting this study as an independent researcher and a volunteer in the healthcare sector.
What am I expected to do?
If you choose to take part in this study, you will be invited to:
Attend four weekly photography workshops, each lasting approximately four hours (including short breaks).

(*Continued*)

TABLE 1.2 (Continued)

PARTICIPANT INFORMATION SHEET
Participate in a one-to-one interview with the researcher, lasting between 90 and 120 minutes.
Take approximately 20 photographs per day that reflect your experiences of managing your illness.
Share and discuss your photographs during the workshops and interview sessions.
Join a two-hour member-checking group at the end of the project to review and provide feedback on the research findings.
Photography training will not be provided as part of this project, so participants are expected to have a basic understanding of photographic techniques. You will need to bring your own equipment – preferably a DSLR camera – to ensure high-quality image capture. Please note that, due to the technical nature of the project, we may not be able to accommodate individuals without prior photography experience or the necessary equipment.
Do I have to take part?
While participation in this study is voluntary, we strongly encourage you to take part due to the valuable insights your extended hospital stay could contribute to the research. You may withdraw at any time during data collection and up to three days following your interview. Choosing not to participate should not affect your access to healthcare services in any way.
Will I be identified in the project?
Your participation will be anonymous, and the information you provide will be treated as confidential, with some limitations, particularly if there is a significant risk of harm to yourself or others. Please note that identifiable data such as faces or locations may be published if deemed highly relevant to the study, and explicit consent for this may not be sought in every case.
What are the benefits of taking part?
While there are no direct personal benefits to participating, you may find the experience enjoyable and rewarding. Your involvement will contribute to improving healthcare services for chronic illness management. Participants who complete all project activities including the interview, four weekly workshops, and the final member-checking group will receive a £200 incentive. Partial participation may not be eligible for compensation.
What are the risks of taking part?
There are no anticipated risks associated with participation. However, if you experience any emotional distress during or after the study, which is highly unlikely, please contact your healthcare provider, as the project does not include any formal debriefing or support services.
What do I need to do next?
If you wish to participate, please complete the consent form as soon as possible and contact the researcher to schedule your initial interview. Workshop dates are fixed and listed in the attached schedule. Attendance is expected for all sessions.
Will my data be kept secure?
Data will be stored on an encrypted, password-protected laptop and backed up on USB sticks. Audio and video recordings will be destroyed after the project is examined. However, anonymised transcripts will be retained indefinitely to allow for publication. Project data may be shared with third parties or used for commercial purposes without prior notice or additional consent.
What if I have questions?
If you have any further questions, feel free to contact me via email, phone, or message me directly on Facebook or Instagram (links provided below).
Thank you for taking the time to read this information sheet!

9.2 Ideas for photography-based research exercises

9.2.1 "I Found Myself in Lost Objects" – expressing experiences of health and illness through photographs of lost objects

Instructions:

Take 3–5 photographs of lost objects found on the street, in the park, or around your home that reflect aspects of your health or illness.

- What do these objects symbolise for you?
- How might they express your health or illness experiences?

Write a short explanation (2–4 sentences) for each photograph.

- Describe the object and where you found it.
- Explain the connection between the object and your health or illness.

Discussion prompts:

- How can apparently ordinary objects become symbols of health or illness experiences?
- Think about your story of health or illness with emphasis on moments of transition, loss, rediscovery, or change in your life.
- Consider how this activity might help you better understand or communicate your journey of health or illness. What insights did you gain through the process?

9.2.2 "Moments That Changed Me" – exploring journeys of transformation and resilience by reenacting a significant moment from the participant's life using photography

Instructions:

- Identify a turning point – think of a moment in your life that marked a change in your health, or perspective on health/illness. This could be a moment of crisis, a revelation, connection, or recovery.
- Reenact the scene – using props, settings, or symbolic elements, recreate the essence of that moment in a set of photographs. You do not need to replicate it literally but try to capture the mood, symbolism, and emotional tone.
- Photograph the reenactment – take 3–5 photos that capture the reenacted moment. You may choose to include yourself, others, or objects that represent your experience.
- Optionally, you may wish to write a short reflection (3–5 sentences) guided by the following questions: What moment did you choose to reenact, and why? How did you decide to visually represent it? What emotions or insights emerged during the process?

Discussion prompts:

- How does reenactment help you process or reframe experiences of health and illness?
- How did reenacting a personal turning point through photography affect your understanding of that experience?

- Did the process of creating the image help you express something that's difficult to put into words? If so, how?

9.2.3 *"A Scene from Our Life" – a group photographic exercise to collaboratively explore shared experiences of living with or supporting someone with a physical or mental health condition through reenacted scenes*

Instructions:

- Each group (3–5 participants) will discuss and identify a common challenge or emotionally significant moment they have experienced in their daily lives (e.g., accessing healthcare, managing symptoms, supporting a loved one).
- As a group, decide how to visually represent this moment. You may choose to reenact it literally or symbolically using props, gestures, or settings. Everyone can contribute ideas and roles.
- Take 2–4 photographs that capture the reenacted moment. You may choose to include people, objects, or settings that convey the emotional tone and context.
- Write a group reflection or narrative guided by the following questions: What moment did you choose to reenact, and why? How did the process of planning and photographing the scene affect your understanding of the experience? What emotions or insights emerged during the activity?

Discussion prompts:

- How did working together influence the way you interpreted and represented the experience?
- Did the reenactment help you see the situation from a new perspective or feel more connected to others in the group?

9.2.4 *"A Life in My Day" – a creative twist on the traditional "A Day in My Life" exercise*

Instead of documenting a chronological routine, this activity invites participants to reflect on how seemingly mundane moments carry emotional, existential, or symbolic meaning, especially in the context of living with, and managing symptoms of, physical illness and/or mental distress.

Instructions:

- Spend some time thinking about what a typical day looks like for you while living with a chronic illness and/or mental distress. Focus on moments that feel emotionally significant, even if they seem mundane, such as making tea, resting, walking, or interacting with others.
- Take 3–5 photographs that represent meaningful aspects of your day. These images might reflect coping strategies or small acts of care and connection. Feel free to use symbols or metaphors to express deeper meanings.
- After capturing your images, reflect (verbally or in writing) on the following prompts: What moments did you choose to represent, and why? How do these moments reflect your experience of living with illness or distress? What do these images reveal about how you cope, find meaning, or maintain well-being?

Discussion prompts:

- How do small, everyday actions help you feel grounded or supported?
- Did this exercise help you see your day differently or discover something meaningful you hadn't noticed before?

9.2.5 "Light and Shadows" (1) – a creative group activity that invites participants to explore the contrasts in, and complexities of, their lived experiences of health and illness

Instructions:

- Begin by discussing the theme of light and shadows in the context of health and illness. What does "light" represent for you? What about "shadows"? Share examples from your daily life that reflect these ideas such as moments of hope, struggle, connection, or solitude.
- Each participant will take 2–3 photographs representing their personal experiences of "light" and "shadow". These could include a comforting routine or a moment of peace ("light"), a space or object that evokes difficulty or uncertainty ("shadow"), or a scene that blends both "light" and "shadow" to illustrate complexity or transition.
- In your group, take turns sharing your photographs and the stories behind them. Use the following prompts to guide your discussion: What does each image represent for you? How do these moments reflect your experience of illness or distress? Did you notice any patterns or contrasts in your own images – or across the group?
- As a group, reflect on the following questions: What did you learn about yourself or others through this process? How do the themes of light and shadow help you understand your experience differently? Were there shared emotions, strategies, or symbols that emerged?

Discussion prompts:

- Did this exercise help you notice something meaningful you hadn't seen before?
- How might these images help others understand what it's like to live with illness or distress?

9.2.6 "Light and Shadows" (2) – adapted to support self-expression, emotional awareness, and shared understanding among people with learning disabilities or cognitive impairments through accessible visual storytelling

Instructions:

- Create a small group (2–4 participants) and include a facilitator or support person, if needed. This activity can be adapted to a one-to-one interview, if this approach works better for the purpose of the study and participants' circumstances.
- Begin with a relaxed conversation about what "light" and "shadow" might mean – happy times, quiet moments, things that feel hard, or things that help. Use visual aids such as printed images, emojis, or drawings to help explain the concepts.

- Each participant takes 1–3 photos using a phone or tablet (with assistance, if needed). These can be something that makes them feel good ("light"), something that feels difficult, confusing, or causes them distress ("shadow"), or a mix of both.
- Participants can point to what they want photographed if they prefer not to take the photo themselves.
- In a group (or one-to-one session), participants share their photos and talk about what they mean. Use prompts like: What is this photo of? How does it make you feel? Is this a light or shadow moment?
- Facilitators can help with communication, using pictures, gestures, or simple words.
- Create a group collage or storybook with the photos and short captions. You can also use emojis, stickers, or drawings to help express feelings.

Discussion prompts:

- What helps you feel better on a shadow day?
- What makes you smile or feel safe?
- Did you learn something new about yourself (or other people in the group)?

9.3 Examples of photographic outputs adaptable to healthcare research

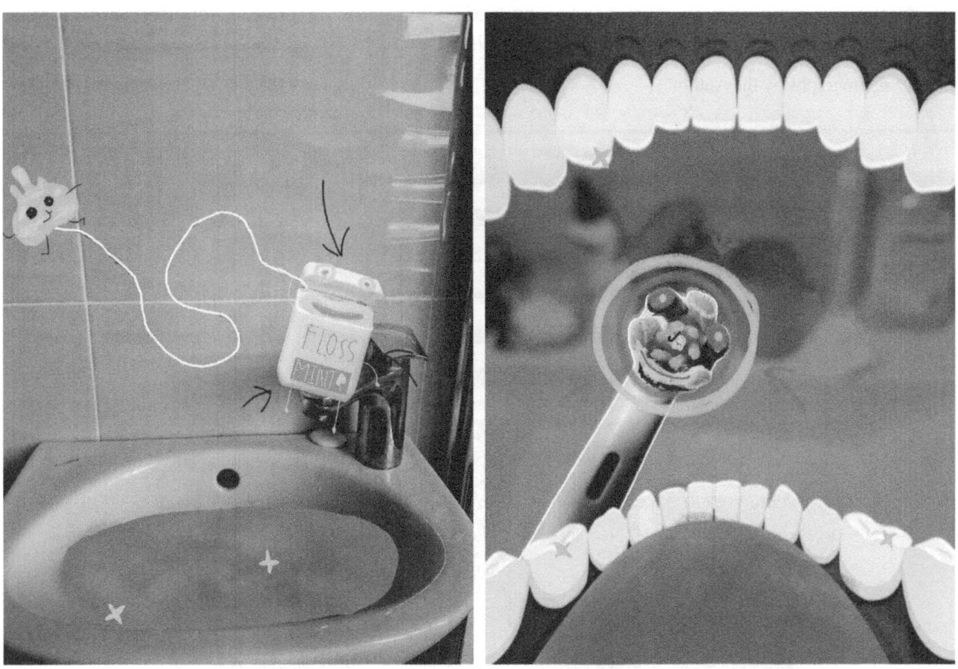

FIGURE 9.2 "Happy teeth" – a creative approach combining photographic imagery with hand-drawn digital illustrations

Source: photographs and illustrations by Nicholas, age 12

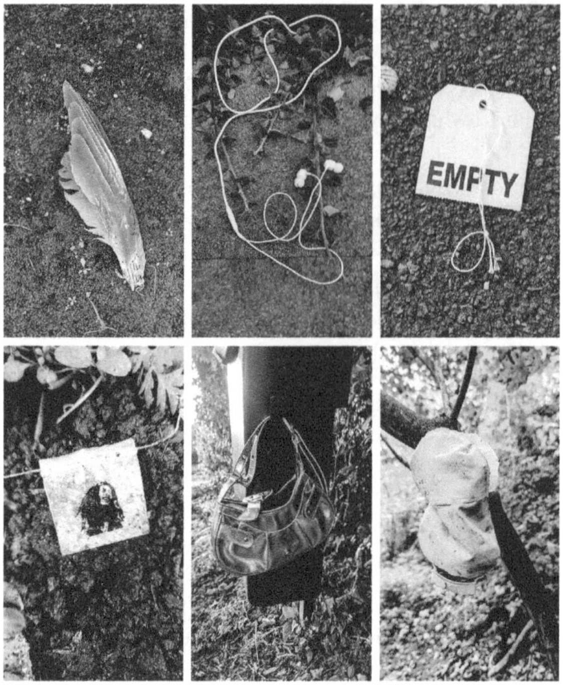

FIGURE 9.3 "Found objects, stories yet to be told" – vignettes for photo-elicitation interviews and focus groups and ice-breaker activities

Source: photographs by the Author

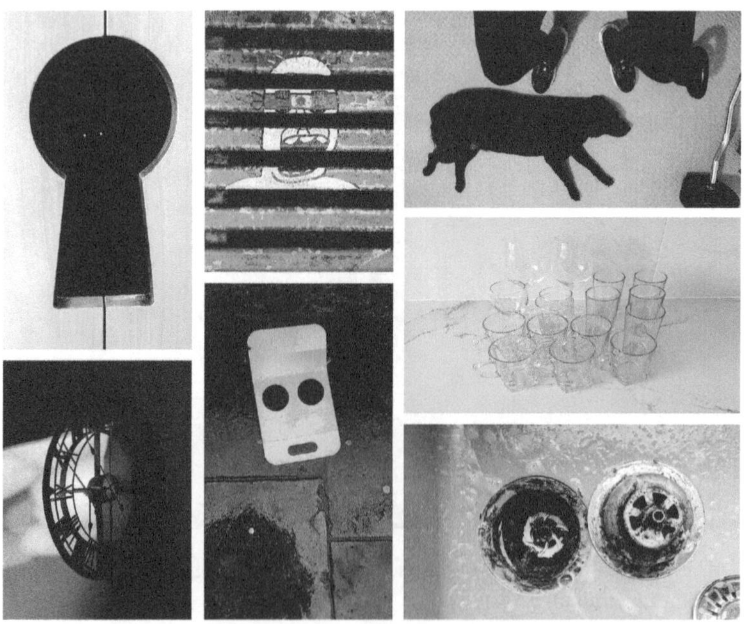

FIGURE 9.4 "A life in a day with depression – a quest for meaning and motivation"

Source: photographs by the Author

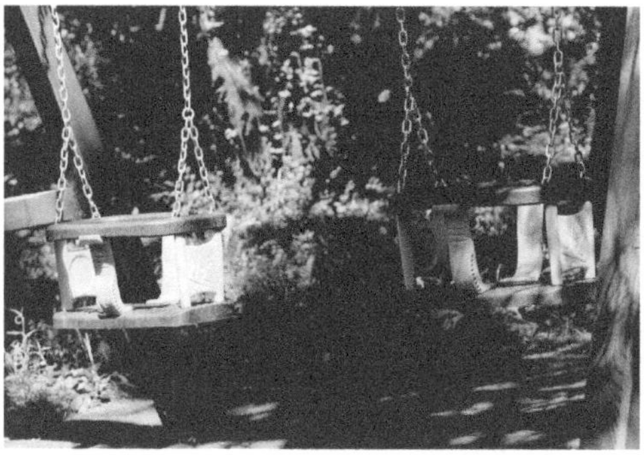

Original image

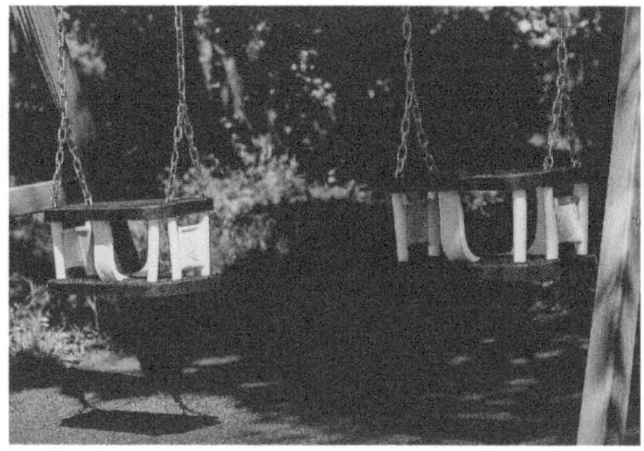

Prompt: Enhance the original image in terms of white balance, exposure, saturation, contrast, and sharpness.

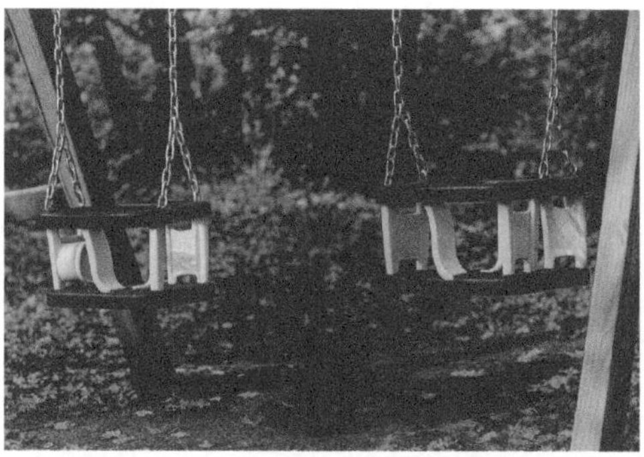

Prompt: Change the original image using warm orange and brown tones, fallen leaves on the ground, and a cozy autumnal atmosphere.

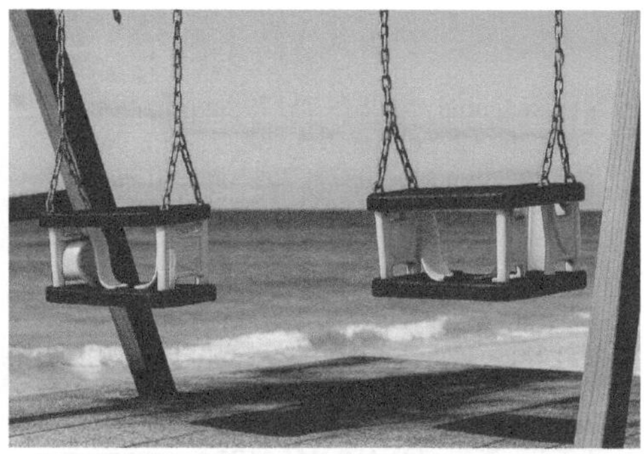

Prompt: Change the scenery to seascape, featuring a clear blue ocean and sandy shore for a bright, coastal feel.

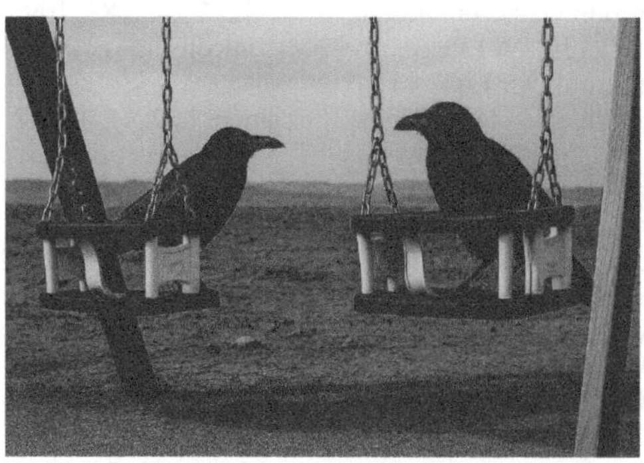

Prompt: Place the swings in a desolate landscape with muted earthy tones and two black crows perched on the seats, to create a dramatic atmosphere.

FIGURE 9.5 Using AI to enhance and recontextualise images

Source: original photograph in top-left corner by Judit; AI imagery generated with Copilot®

INDEX

For Product Safety Concerns and Information please contact our EU representative GPSR@taylorandfrancis.com Taylor & Francis Verlag GmbH, Kaufingerstraße 24, 80331 München, Germany